ECG Interpretation in the Critically Ill Dog and Cat

ECG Interpretation in the Critically Ill Dog and Cat

Thomas K. Day, DVM, MS, DACVA, DACVECC

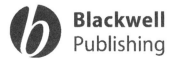

Blackwell Publishing

Thomas K. Day received his DVM from The Ohio State University. Dr. Day is a Diplomate of the American College of Veterinary Anesthesiologists and a Diplomate of the American College of Veterinary Emergency and Critical Care. Dr. Day presently practices at Louisville Veterinary Specialty and Emergency Services, Louisville, Kentucky.

Blackwell Publishing Professional
2121 State Avenue, Ames, Iowa 50014, USA

Orders: 1-800-862-6657
Office: 1-515-292-0140
Fax: 1-515-292-3348
Web site: www.blackwellprofessional.com

Blackwell Publishing Ltd
9600 Garsington Road, Oxford OX4 2DQ, UK
Tel.: +44 (0)1865 776868

Blackwell Publishing Asia
550 Swanston Street, Carlton, Victoria 3053, Australia
Tel.: +61 (0)3 8359 1011

First edition, 2005

Library of Congress Cataloging-in-Publication Data
Day, Thomas K., 1960–
    ECG interpretation in the critically ill dog and cat /
    Thomas K. Day.
      p. cm.
    Includes index.
    ISBN-13: 978-0-8138-0901-4 (alk. paper)
    ISBN-10: 0-8138-0901-0 (alk. paper)
    1. Dogs—Diseases—Diagnosis.   2. Cats—Diseases—
    Diagnosis.   3. Veterinary electrocardiography.   4. Critical
care medicine.   I. Title.

SF992.C37.D39 2005
636.7′0896075—dc22   2005005244

Printed and bound by CPI Group (UK) Ltd, Croydon, CR0 4YY

C9780813809014_181024

Dedication

This book is dedicated to all of the past, present and future students, technicians, interns, residents, practitioners, and colleagues who provided encouragement and support for this project. The vast majority of the case presentations in this book arrived from patients in the ICU or on the emergency room floor during the training of future clinicians. The inspiration to write this book is certainly all of the students and veterinarians I have and will encounter. However, the completion of this book is entirely dedicated to my wife, Deborah, who has provided support and enduring love that words are unable to describe.

Contents

Renal

Trauma

Preface

There are many excellent textbooks that provide detailed information on how to interpret the electrocardiogram (ECG). You are encouraged to study these texts to acquire a base knowledge of the normal ECG and the various types of ECG abnormalities. This text was designed to emphasize ECG abnormalities based on case presentations and the indications to perform an ECG. The ECG can then be interpreted based on the abnormalities of the patient and the influence of disease process on the cardiac conduction system.

You will find that the emphasis on therapy for an ECG abnormality may not necessarily involve the use of antiarrhythmic drugs. Therefore, the reader of this book will be able to gain knowledge of the multitude of causes of ECG abnormalities, as well as the ability to recognize all possible therapeutic interventions, including antiarrhythmic drugs.

How to Use This Book

The electrocardiograms (ECGs) presented in this book represent a diagnostic "piece" of information regarding the status of the cardiac conduction system in dogs or cats. A brief case is presented with pertinent information needed to provide an assessment of the ECG that follows the case on the same page. You are asked to make the ECG diagnosis and provide therapy for the patient that will correct the ECG abnormality. The ECG interpretation and approaches to therapy of the patient and the ECG begin on the following page. You will benefit the most by providing the best answer possible prior to looking at the answer that follows the case presentation. Each case is presented in a random fashion, with no regard to the type of ECG abnormality. The categories of disease processes that can result in an ECG abnormality have been organized in a general fashion without the presentation of a diagnosis.

Note: All ECG tracings are lead II, and the paper speed is 25 mm/s with 1 mV equal to 10 mm (1 cm).

Continuous monitoring of the ECG during anesthesia or during hospitalization can provide the clinician with valuable information that may be missed with intermittent ECG monitoring. There are many manufacturers of ECG monitors including bedside monitors (Figure FM.1) and telemetry units (Figure FM.2). Telemetry units afford the advantage of continuous ECG evaluation without having the ECG monitor near the cage. Most telemetry units can detect the ECG up to 1000 feet from the main monitor.

Knowledge of the normal P-QRS-T complex is essential to determine abnormal ECG complexes.

The normal ECG in the dog consists of the P-wave, P-R interval, QRS complex, T-wave, and Q-T interval (Figure FM3).

The P-wave represents electrical conduction from the sinus node to the atrioventricular (AV) node. Discharge from the sinus node is synonymous with the sinus rate.

The P-R interval represents conduction through the AV node. Conduction through the AV node is the rate-limiting, or slowest, conduction within the cardiac electrical system.

The QRS complex represents conduction from the AV node, through the Bundle of His and through the ventricle via the Purkinje fibers. The R-wave is positive in lead II of the ECG.

The T-wave represents repolarization of the ventricle and can be positive, negative, or biphasic.

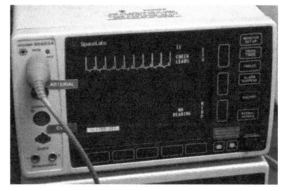

Figure FM.1. Bedside ECG monitor.

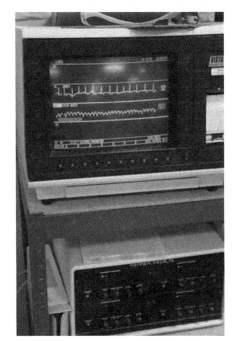

Figure FM.2. Telemetry unit.

The Q-T interval represents the relative time of ventricular repolarization.

The normal sinus discharge in dogs depends somewhat on size of the dog. Small dogs (< 5 kg) have normal sinus rates of 100–140 bpm. Large dogs (> 30 kg) have a normal sinus rate of 80–100 bpm.

The intrinsic rate of the ventricle in dogs is 40–80 bpm.

The normal feline ECG has several differences compared to the canine ECG (Figure FM.4). The rate of sinus node discharge is more rapid, and the QRS complexes are relatively smaller. The same electric physiology that occurs in the canine occurs in the feline. The intrinsic sinus node discharge rate is 160–200 bpm. The intrinsic ventricular discharge rate is 130–150 bpm.

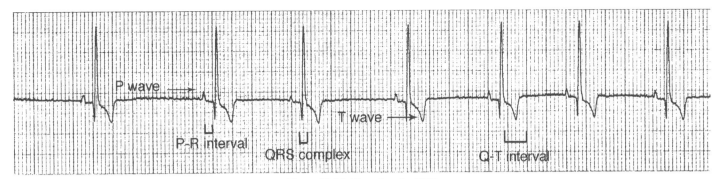

Figure FM.3. Normal canine ECG.

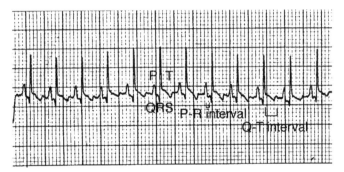

Figure FM.4. Normal feline ECG.

Anesthesia

Case 1

A healthy 3-year-old M Wiemaraner (30 kg) has been sedated with acepromazine (0.05 mg/kg, IV) and hydromorphone (0.1 mg/kg, IV) to repair a laceration on the right forelimb. A local anesthetic (lidocaine, 5 ml) has been infiltrated around the wound. The heart rate has decreased, and the mucous membranes are pale. An ECG is performed.

Describe the arrhythmia or conduction disturbance and your approach to therapy. The answer and discussion appear on the next page.

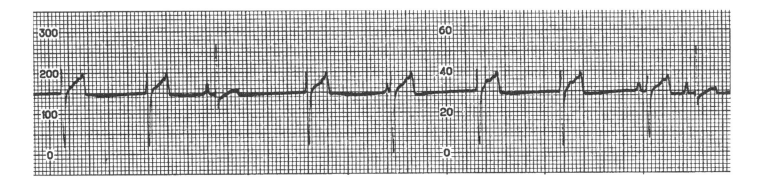

Interpretation

The rhythm is sinus bradycardia (60 bpm) with a ventricular escape rhythm. A normal P-QRS-T complex occurs in the middle of the rhythm strip (thin arrow). The intrinsic ventricular rate in the dog is 40–60 bpm. A ventricular escape rhythm occurs when there is a delay in ventricular conduction from the sinus node. The primary cause of the rhythm in this dog is likely increased parasympathetic tone induced by the opioid agonist hydromorphone. A parasympatholytic agent such as atropine (0.02 mg/kg, IV) or glycopyrrolate (0.025 mg/kg, IV) can be administered to increase the rate of sinus node discharge, which will eliminate the ventricular escape rhythm. The decision to administer the atropine or glycopyrrolate is not necessarily based on the ECG, but on whether perfusion is being compromised. The clinical finding of pale mucous membranes indicates that perfusion has decreased and that a parasympatholytic agent is indicated. An antiarrhythmic agent such as lidocaine or procainamide will eliminate the ventricular escape rhythm and is therefore contraindicated.

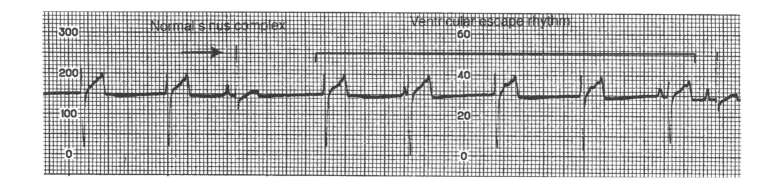

Case 2

An 8-month-old F Labrador (25 kg) is anesthetized for an ovario-hysterectomy. Acepromazine (0.05 mg/kg, IM) and butorphanol (0.2 mg/kg, IM) were administered as preanesthetic medication, propofol (4 mg/kg, IV) was administered as the induction agent, and sevoflurane is the inhalation anesthetic. An esophageal ECG is used to monitor the heart rate and rhythm. The technician alerts you that the ECG looks abnormal. Mucous membranes are pink and the lingual pulse is strong. Indirect blood pressure is normal.

Describe the arrhythmia or conduction disturbance and your approach to therapy. The answer and discussion appear on the next page.

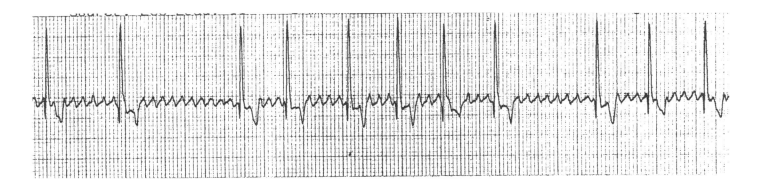

Interpretation

The rhythm disturbance is atrial flutter with irregular conduction to the ventricle. There are numerous P-waves that occur in a regular pattern between each normal QRS complex. The ventricular complexes occur at an irregular rate due to the limited conduction through the atrioventricular (AV) node. Atrial flutter can occur as a tachyarrhythmia when the AV nodal conduction is normal. The influence of anesthetic agents on the AV node is an explanation as to why the ventricular rate is not rapid. The overall ventricular rate (90 bpm) is not affected by the atrial flutter. There is no therapy for atrial flutter, as spontaneous resolution usually occurs (star, lower figure).

Normal sinus rhythm occurs following atrial flutter (following page). The overall ventricular rate (70 bpm) is slower than during atrial flutter but is still considered normal in this dog and does not require therapy.

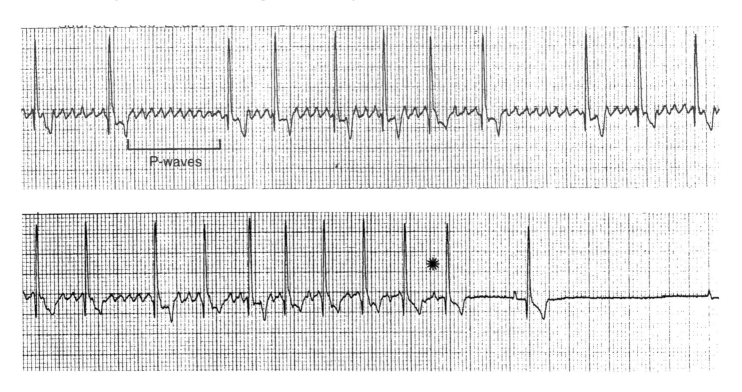

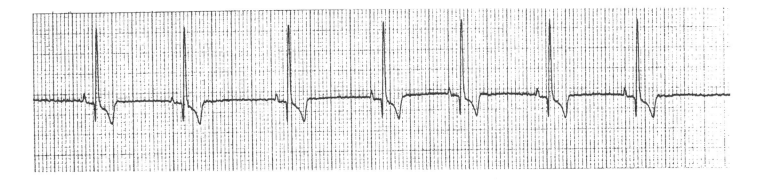

Case 3

A 6-month-old F Yorkshire terrier (3 kg) is anesthetized for an ovariohysterectomy. Preanesthetic medication consisted of diazepam (0.2 mg/kg, IM) and butorphanol (0.4 mg/kg, IM), induction was with propofol (4 mg/kg, IV), and maintenance is with isoflurane. The technician notifies you that the heart rate has dropped to 80 bpm, and the indirect systolic blood pressure is 80 mmHg. A dose of atropine (0.02 mg/kg. IM) is administered. The technician reports that the heart rate is now 70 bpm, and the ECG appears abnormal.

Describe the arrhythmia or conduction disturbance and your approach to therapy. The answer and discussion appear on the next page.

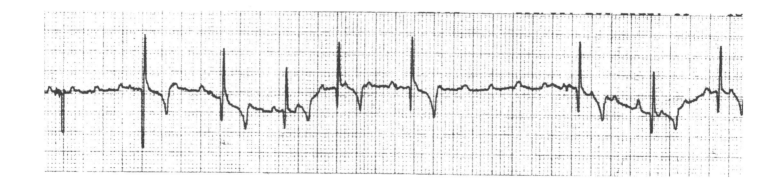

Interpretation

The ECG shows an accelerated sinus response noted by P-waves that are not followed by QRS complexes. The normal P-QRS-T complex is a first-degree atrioventricular (AV) block that is indicated by the prolonged P-R interval. There are two possible explanations for the increased sinus node discharge without a concurrent increase in ventricular activity. One is that there is more blood flow to the sinus node relative to the AV node and the atropine affects the sinus node before the AV node, resulting in relatively more P-waves than concurrent QRS complexes. The second is that there may be more parasympathetic innervation to the AV node, which will result in the same imbalance between P-waves and QRS complexes. Regardless of the cause, bradycardia may occur before the increased normal sinus rhythm. The primary therapy is to wait for several minutes and not administer more atropine.

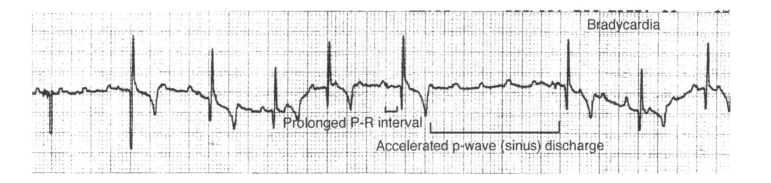

Case 4

A 6-month-old F domestic shorthair cat (3.5 kg) is anesthetized for an ovariohysterectomy and front onychectomy. Anesthesia consists of ketamine (15 mg/kg), acepromazine (0.1 mg/kg), and butorphanol (0.2 mg/kg), all administered IM prior to induction of anesthesia with propofol (4 mg/kg, IV). The cat is receiving isoflurane in oxygen. The doppler begins to sound erratic as the ovary is manipulated, and the systolic blood pressure increases to 150 mmHg. The jaw tone is tense and the cat begins to move. The ECG becomes erratic as well.

Describe the arrhythmia or conduction disturbance and your approach to therapy. The answer and discussion appear on the next page.

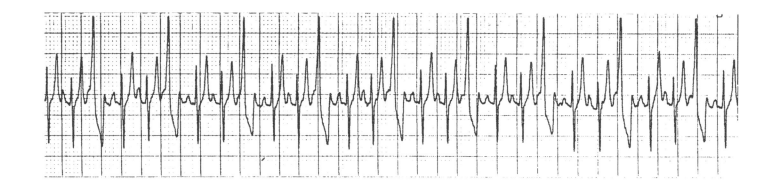

Interpretation

The rhythm diagnosis is sinus tachycardia with premature ventricular complexes (thick arrows). The sinus complexes (circles) can easily be overlooked when the heart rate is so rapid. The most likely cause of the arrhythmia is inadequate anesthetic depth resulting in an increase in catecholamine release secondary to pain. The primary therapy is to temporarily discontinue surgical stimulation while the depth of anesthesia is increased, by increasing the amount of isoflurane and/or administration of a more potent analgesic agent such as hydromorphone (0.1 mg/kg, IV). Antiarrhythmic therapy may not be warranted, based on the results of increasing anesthetic depth and providing additional analgesia.

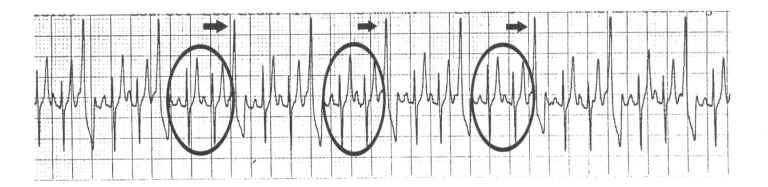

Case 5

A 10-year-old F Poodle (5 kg) has been diagnosed with pyometra and surgery is underway. All chemistries were within normal limits, and fluid therapy had been administered for several hours, including hetastarch and lactated Ringer's solution (LRS) with potassium supplementation. Diazepam (0.2 mg/kg, IV) and hydromorphone (0.1 mg/kg, IV) were administered prior to anesthetic induction with ketamine and diazepam (1 ml of a 50:50 mixture/10 kg). Maintenance anesthesia is with isoflurane and oxygen. An ECG and doppler have been in place since induction. Shortly after induction, you notice that the doppler rate suddenly decreases.

Describe the arrhythmia or conduction disturbance and your approach to therapy. The answer and discussion appear on the next page.

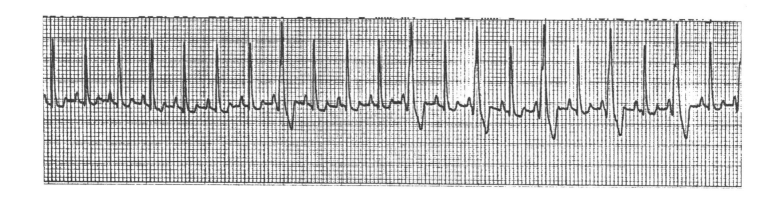

Interpretation

The initial rhythm is sinus tachycardia. Premature ventricular complexes (arrows) occur in a bigeminal pattern. The presence of P-waves preceding the premature ventricular complexes (PVCs) is of no consequence. The sinus node and the abnormal QRS complex have discharged prior to the continuation of the sinus electrical activity to the ventricle. Anesthetic depth must be assessed and blood pressure determined to decide whether or not an antiarrhythmic agent is required.

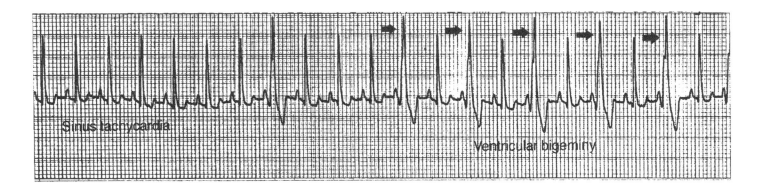

Case 6

A 16-year-old FS domestic shorthair cat (6 kg) presents for evaluation of chronic vomiting and an endoscopy is scheduled. Physical examination is unremarkable. Thoracic auscultation is unremarkable, and the heart rate is 150 bpm. A preoperative ECG is performed and evaluated as normal.

The cat is anesthetized with diazepam (0.4 mg/kg) and butorphanol (0.2 mg/kg) administered IV prior to propofol (5 mg/kg,

IV) and placed on isoflurane. The heart rate drops dramatically, hypotension occurs, and the ECG is reexamined (ECG, page 15).

Describe the arrhythmia or conduction disturbance and your approach to therapy. The answer and discussion appear on page 16.

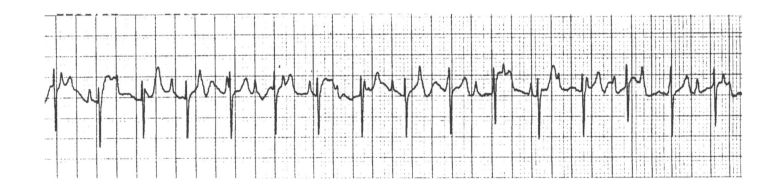

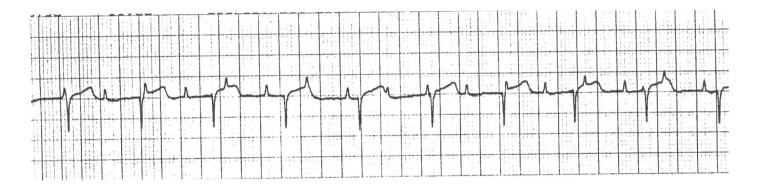

Interpretation

The rhythm is a third-degree or complete atrioventricular (AV) block. The sinus node discharge is normal (165 bpm) and is represented by the P-waves (thin lines). The ventricular rate is slow (80 bpm) and has no association with the P-waves (thick lines). The hypotension results in termination of the procedure, and anesthesia is discontinued.

Reexamination of the initial ECG reveals a third-degree block as well (lower figure). The sinus rate is rapid (200 bpm), yet the ventricular rate is slower (150 bpm). There is no association between the P-waves and QRS complexes.

Third-degree AV block can be a spontaneous occurrence in cats. However, an echocardiogram is indicated to investigate the possibility of primary heart disease.

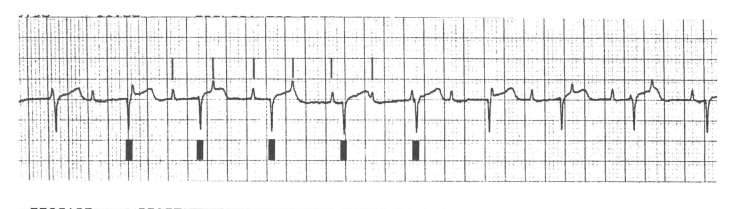

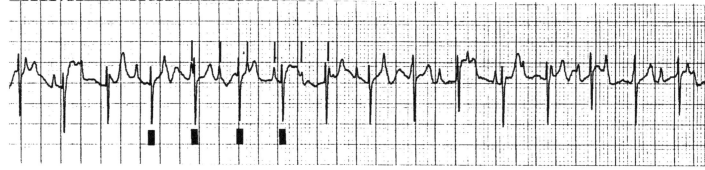

Case 7

A 2-year-old M mixed-breed dog (10 kg) presents with a non–weight-bearing lameness of the front right limb. The owners are unsure of the cause, though the dog runs in their 3/4-acre, fenced-in yard with the other family dog, which is much larger. Physical examination is difficult due to severe pain. You are able to confirm normal thoracic auscultation. You decide to administer medetomidine (0.02 mg/kg) and hydromorphone (0.1 mg/kg), both administered IM. The mucous membranes become pale, the heart rate is slow, and the pulse is weak. An ECG is performed.

Describe the arrhythmia or conduction disturbance and your approach to therapy. The answer and discussion appear on the next page.

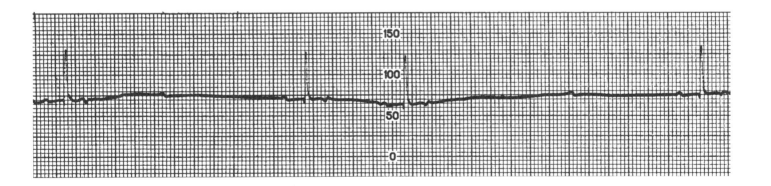

Interpretation

The rhythm is sinus bradycardia (thin lines), and the ventricular rate is slow (40 bpm) and irregular. There are two conduction disturbances. The P-R interval is prolonged (bars), which defines a first-degree atrioventricular (AV) block. There are P-waves with no QRS complex (thick lines), which defines a second-degree AV block. The likely cause of the bradycardia and the conduction disturbances is the combination of medetomidine and hydromor-phone. Both anesthetic drugs increase parasympathetic tone, which will decrease sinus node discharge (bradycardia) and slow conduction through the AV node (first- and second-degree AV block). Therapy would consist of atropine administration (0.02 mg/kg, IV) or reversal of medetomidine with atipamezole (same volume as medetomidine, IM) and/or reversal of hydromorphone with naloxone (0.04 mg/kg, IV). Reversal of both anesthetic drugs will result in the reversal of the effects of the analgesia.

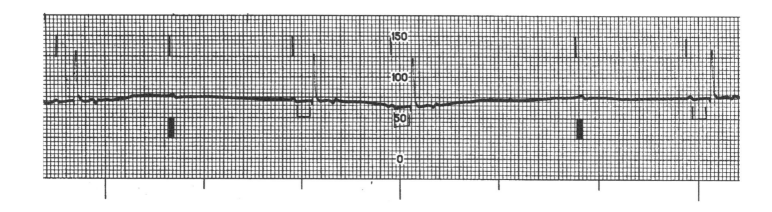

Case 8

A 3-year-old MN domestic shorthair cat (3.5 kg) is anesthetized for removal of a gastric foreign object. The physical examination and laboratory parameters were within normal limits. Anesthesia consists of diazepam (0.3 mg/kg) and butorphanol (0.2 mg/kg) IV prior to induction with propofol (4 mg/kg, IV) and maintenance with isoflurane in oxygen. The doppler blood pressure is normal, yet the ECG appears unusual.

Describe the arrhythmia or conduction disturbance and your approach to therapy. The answer and discussion appear on the next page.

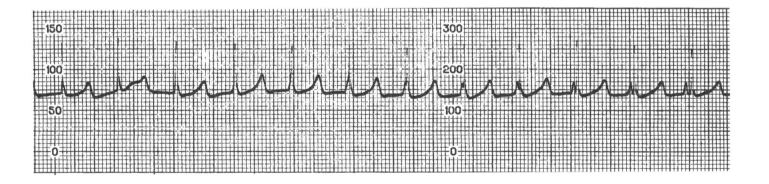

Interpretation

The arrhythmia is isorhythmic atrioventricular dissociation (nodal tachycardia), which is common with isoflurane anesthesia. The ventricular rate is slightly lower than normal (110 bpm), and the QRS complexes are normal. The sinus rate is also near normal (110 bpm) and is similar to the ventricular rate (thin lines). There is no association between the P-waves and the QRS complexes. In fact, the P-waves appear to move in and out of the QRS complexes. The ventricular rate is likely a ventricular arrhythmia that has originated high in the ventricle, resulting in a normal QRS complex. The blood pressure is normal, and the overall ventricular rate is acceptable for an anesthetized cat. No antiarrhythmic therapy or alteration of anesthetic depth is indicated. The arrhythmia resolves after anesthesia.

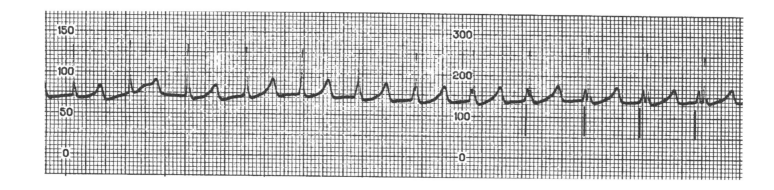

Cardiovascular

Case 9

An 11-year-old FS Cornish Rex cat (4 kg) presents in respiratory distress. Thoracic auscultation reveals muffled lung sounds ventrally, though lung sounds can be heard dorsally. The heart sounds are muffled. Pleural effusion is diagnosed. A total of 175 ml of chylous effusion is removed via thoracocentesis, and an echocardio-gram reveals dilated cardiomyopathy. The heart rate is slow and regular. An ECG is performed.

Describe the arrhythmia or conduction disturbance and your approach to therapy. The answer and discussion appear on the next page.

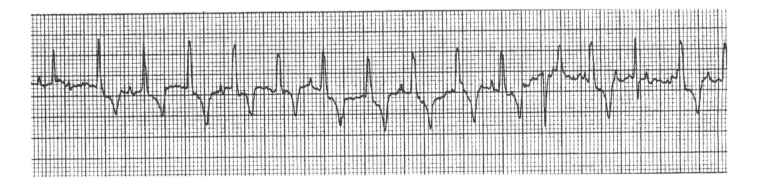

Interpretation

The ECG diagnosis is third-degree atrioventricular (AV) block. P-waves (thin lines) occasionally appear throughout the rhythm strip and have no association with the ventricular complexes. The sinus rate (P-waves) is normal at 180 bpm. The ventricular complexes originate from three different foci within the ventricle (thick arrows), as determined by three different shapes of the QRS complex. The ventricular rate is 140 bpm and regular. The ventricular rhythm is an escape rhythm that occurs when no electrical activity enters the ventricle from the sinus node. The intrinsic ventricular rate of the feline ventricle is 130–150 bpm. The ventricular complexes are not premature in origin, and lidocaine or other antiarrhythmic therapy is not indicated. Administration of an antiarrhythmic agent could result in elimination of any ventricular activity and death of the cat. Definitive therapy for third-degree AV block is placement of a ventricular pacemaker.

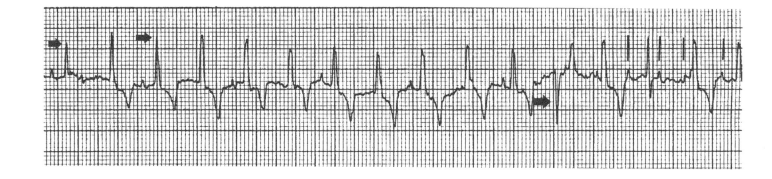

Case 10

A 6-year-old MN Scottish deerhound (45 kg) presents for evaluation of lethargy and exercise intolerance. Physical examination reveals a grade 3/6 systolic apical heart murmur that is most prominent at the ventral left hemithorax. The heart rate is rapid and irregular. The femoral pulses are weak and irregular with pulse deficits. There are mild crackles, bilaterally, and slightly muffled heart sounds. Thoracic radiography reveals hilar pulmonary edema, mild pleural effusion, and generalized cardiomegaly. Dilated cardiomyopathy is diagnosed via echocardiography. An ECG is performed.

Describe the arrhythmia or conduction disturbance and your approach to therapy. The answer and discussion appear on the next page.

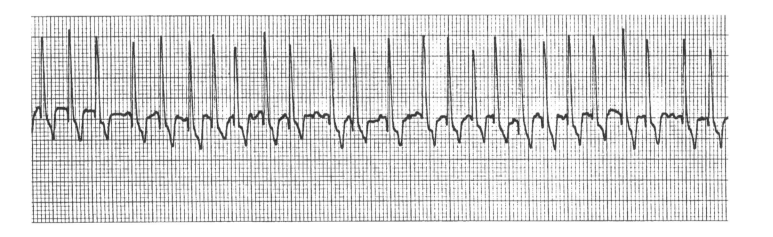

Interpretation

The ECG rhythm diagnosis is atrial fibrillation. Criteria for atrial fibrillation include a rapid, irregular ventricular rate, normal QRS complexes, lack of P-waves, and the presence of fibrillation waves (f-waves). F-waves (thin lines) occur instead of P-waves as sinus node discharge has been replaced by chaotic atrial conduction. The QRS complexes are normal in appearance and occur in a rapid, irregular rhythm (240 bpm). Fibrillation of the atria results in constant electric stimulation of the atrioventricular (AV) node. The AV node conducts electrical activity to the ventricle in a rapid, irregular pattern, resulting in normal, rapid, and irregular QRS complexes. Therapy for cardiogenic failure (furosemide, 2 mg/kg, IV; digoxin; and enalapril, 0.25 mg/kg, PO BID) is instituted. Digoxin is the initial drug of choice for atrial fibrillation. Digoxin slows conduction through the AV node, resulting in slower discharge to the ventricle and a reduced ventricular rate. A loading dose of digoxin can be administered orally. The daily dose of digoxin is 0.22 mg/m^2 (body surface area) twice daily. The conversion from kilograms to body surface area must be made prior to dose calculation and administration of the digoxin. If the dog's body surface area is 1.25 m^2, the daily dose is approximately 0.5 mg. The entire calculated daily dose (0.55 mg) should be administered twice on the first day of therapy. The dose of digoxin can then be administered at the appropriate dose (0.25 mg) twice daily on the second day.

The congestion has resolved 48 hours later, and the femoral pulse rate is slower than on presentation.

A second ECG is performed (next page).

The ventricular rate has decreased to near normal (100 bpm) and remains irregular. The f-waves are more evident as the ventricular rate decreases.

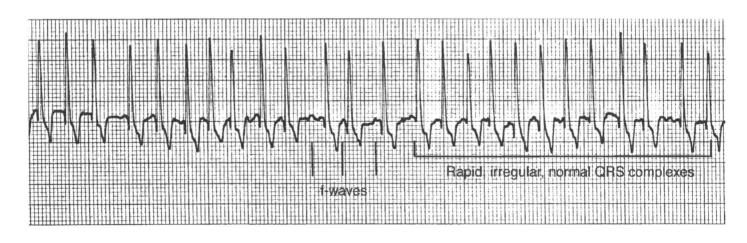

f-waves

Rapid, irregular, normal QRS complexes

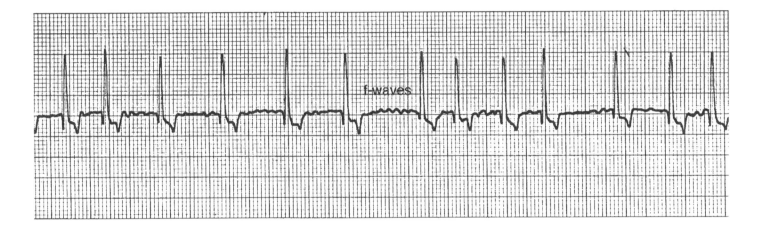

Case 11

A 9-year-old FS Siamese presents for multiple syncopal episodes. Physical examination is unremarkable except for a very slow and regular heart rate and femoral pulse rate with no pulse deficits. Thoracic auscultation reveals a 3/6 systolic murmur, heard best at the left apex, and normal lung sounds. Echocardiography reveals bilateral atrial enlargement and dilated, poorly contracting ventri-cles. The diagnosis of dilated cardiomyopathy is made. An ECG is performed.

Describe the arrhythmia or conduction disturbance and your approach to therapy. The answer and discussion appear on the next page.

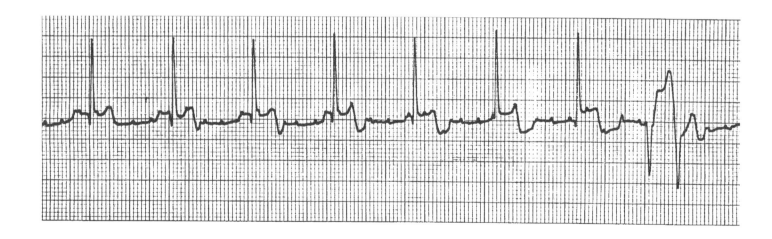

Interpretation

The rhythm indicates a third-degree or complete atrioventricular (AV) block. The line graph demonstrates the lack of association between P-waves (short lines) and QRS complexes (long lines). The small lines represent normal discharge of the sinus node (250 bpm). The large lines demonstrate the intrinsic ventricular rate for the cat (70–130 bpm). The cat clinically is not in congestive heart failure. Definitive therapy would consist of a ventricular pacemaker.

There are two ventricular complexes with R-on-T phenomena (circle). The ventricular complexes originate from a different site within the ventricle because the shape of the QRS complex is different than that of the ventricular escape complexes. These likely developed as a result of poor perfusion to the ventricular myocardium because of the heart disease. Administration of an antiarrhythmic agent such as lidocaine to control the R-on-T is not recommended. Lidocaine will result in termination of the ventricular escape rhythm. Laboratory tests should commence to determine if there is another cause of the ventricular arrhythmia (hypokalemia, hypercalcemia, etc.). The R-on-T phenomenon is not a contraindication to placement of a pacemaker. Medical therapy for the dilated cardiomyopathy would include a positive inotrope such as digoxin.

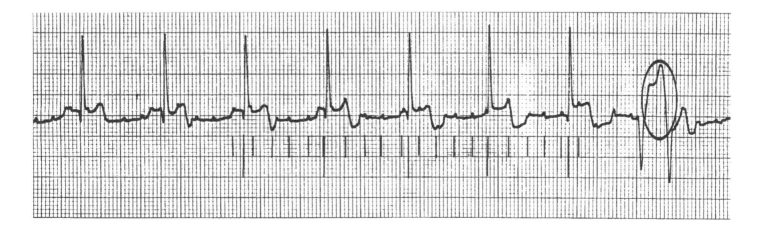

Case 12

A 7-year-old MN Great Dane mix (35 kg) presents for lethargy and exercise intolerance. Physical examination reveals a very lethargic dog. Thoracic auscultation reveals a very rapid, irregular heart rate with no cardiac murmur. Femoral pulses are weak, rapid, and irregular with many pulse deficits. An ECG is performed.

Describe the arrhythmia or conduction disturbance and your immediate approach to therapy. The answer and discussion appear on the following pages.

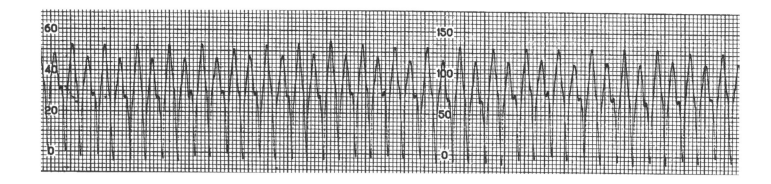

Initial Interpretation

The rhythm diagnosis is sustained ventricular tachycardia with a rate of 360 bpm. The specific term for this type of sustained ventricular tachycardia is torsade de pointes.

The primary cause of the lethargy and exercise intolerance is likely the extremely high ventricular rate, as there are no clinical signs of congestive heart failure. Immediate cessation of the rhythm is indicated. An IV catheter is placed in a cephalic vein. Li-docaine (2 mg/kg, IV) is administered as a slow bolus. Other options include procainamide (6 mg/kg, IV, over 5 minutes) and magnesium sulfate (30 mg/kg, IV). The ECG (lower figure) appears to have converted out of sustained ventricular tachycardia.

Describe the arrhythmia or conduction disturbance and your approach to therapy. The answer and discussion appear on the next page.

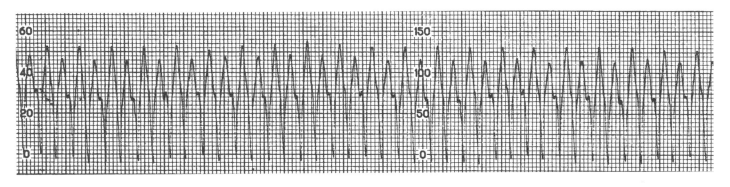

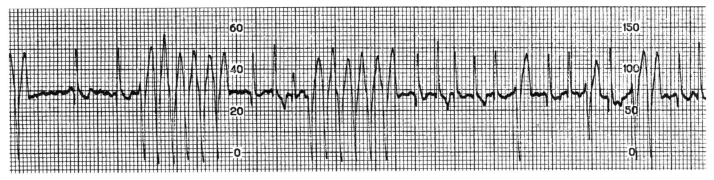

Follow-up Interpretation

The rhythm diagnosis is paroxysmal ventricular tachycardia with R-on-T phenomena (circle). There is a second arrhythmia in the ECG that is atrial fibrillation. Considerations for therapy of both ventricular and supraventricular arrhythmias include calcium channel antagonists (diltiazem) and beta-blockers (atenolol). Other considerations include digoxin to treat the atrial fibrillation and oral procainamide or sotalol to help control the ventricular arrhythmias. An echocardiogram provides the diagnosis of dilated cardiomyopathy.

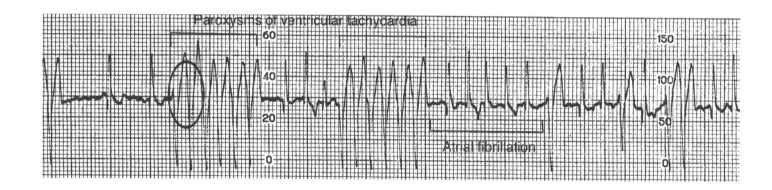

Case 13

A 15-year-old MN domestic longhair cat presents in respiratory distress. The history is unremarkable. Thoracic auscultation reveals bilateral fine crackles and a grade 4/6 systolic murmur, heard loudest at the left apex. The femoral pulse rate is very erratic, and there are pulse deficits. You perform an ECG during initial therapy of oxygen administration.

Describe the arrhythmia or conduction disturbance and your approach to therapy. The answer and discussion appear on the next page.

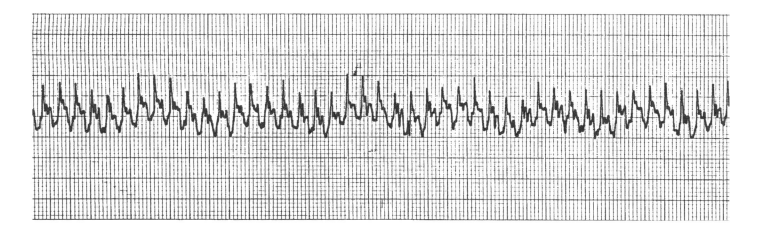

Initial Interpretation

The rhythm is rapid (360 bpm) and regular. The QRS complexes appear to be normal in width and may be supraventricular in origin. However, it is difficult to determine if the rhythm is supraventricular or ventricular as the rate is too rapid and there is no normal P-QRS-T complex for comparison. Therapy is initiated with furosemide (2 mg/kg, IM) and nitroglycerine paste (1/4 inch transdermally). The cat is able to have an echocardiogram, which reveals hypertrophic cardiomyopathy with enlargement of the left atrium. The respiratory distress resolves with medical therapy in 24 hours and the ECG is reexamined (page 35).

Describe the arrhythmia or conduction disturbance and your approach to therapy. The answer and discussion appear on the following pages.

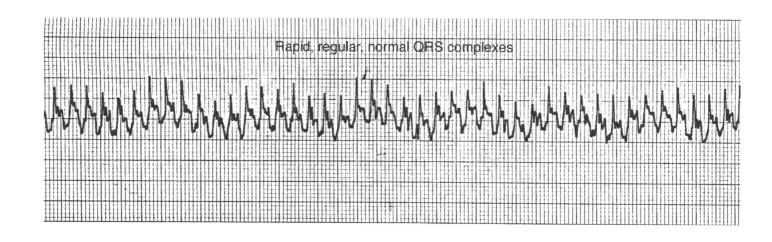

Rapid, regular, normal QRS complexes

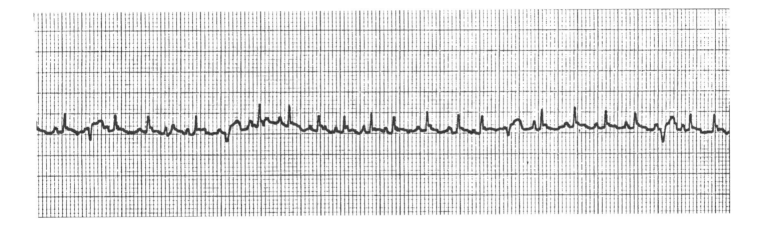

Follow-up Interpretation

The rhythm diagnosis is normal sinus rhythm with occasional ventricular premature complexes (circles). The QRS complexes of the initial ECG are similar to those of the normal QRS complexes. Therefore, the initial ECG diagnosis is supraventricular tachycardia. The decision to institute antiarrhythmic therapy on initial presentation is usually determined after congestion is relieved. Diltiazem is a calcium channel antagonist that is a recommended therapy for cats with hypertrophic cardiomyopathy. Diltiazem could also be used to control supraventricular tachycardia.

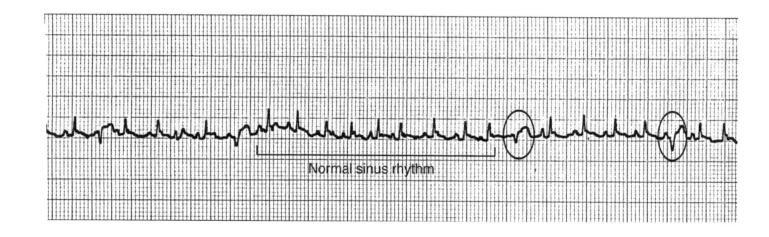

Normal sinus rhythm

Case 14

A 14-year-old FS Beagle (10 kg) is presented for evaluation of acute respiratory distress. She has been treated for mitral insufficiency for the last 4 years and is currently receiving enalapril. The dog acutely went into respiratory distress after running through the house. Physical examination reveals fulminate pulmonary edema (pink, foamy fluid from the nostrils and bilateral fine crackles), a grade 5/6 systolic murmur heard loudest over the left hemithorax, and a very weak and rapid femoral pulse. An ECG is performed while acute cardiogenic failure therapy is instituted with furosemide (2 mg/kg, IV) and nitroglycerine (1/4 inch transdermally).

Describe the arrhythmia or conduction disturbance and your approach to therapy. The answer and discussion appear on the next page.

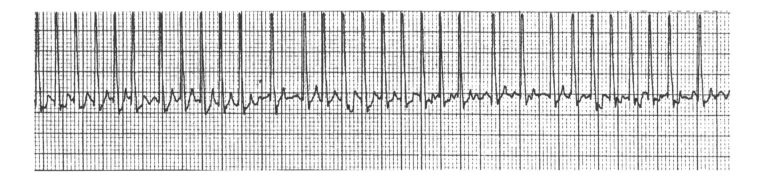

Interpretation

The rhythm diagnosis is atrial fibrillation. The QRS complexes are normal in appearance, rapid, and irregular. There is no consistent R-R interval (bars), and there are no discernible P-waves. Rapid atrial fibrillation can be mistaken for supraventricular tachycardia (normal appearance of QRS complexes, rapid and regular rate). Acute decompensation to congestive heart failure after several years of normal activity can be caused by chordae tendinae rupture or development of an arrhythmia. Acute onset of atrial fibrillation or supraventricular tachycardia can result in acute decompensation in dogs with mitral valve disease. Acute therapy for the arrhythmia could consist of digitalis glycosides (oral-loading dose or intravenous administration) or calcium channel blockers (verapamil, 0.5 mg/kg, IV; diltiazem, 0.1 mg/kg, IV, over 5 minutes).

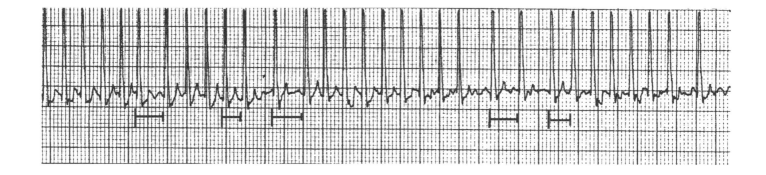

Case 15

A 6-year-old MN domestic shorthair cat (6 kg) presents in acute respiratory distress. Pleural effusion has been identified, and 200 ml of a transudate has been removed. Thoracic auscultation reveals a very irregular heart rhythm with corresponding pulse deficits. You perform an ECG as part of your diagnostics plan.

Describe the arrhythmia or conduction disturbance and your approach to therapy. The answer and discussion appear on the following pages.

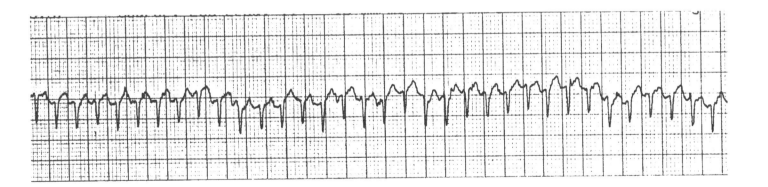

Initial Interpretation

The initial rhythm diagnosis is ventricular tachycardia. The QRS complexes are wide and bizarre, and the ventricular rate is regular.

Increasing the paper speed to 50 mm/s can be helpful in determining if P-waves are present (lower figure).

More discussion and ECG on the next page.

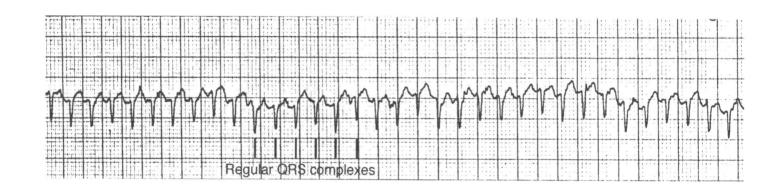

Regular QRS complexes

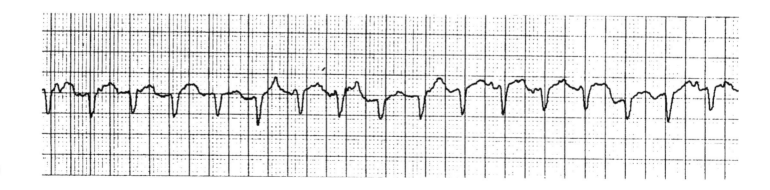

Follow-up Interpretation

P-waves are identified (short vertical lines), which indicates that the sinus node has function. Identification of P-waves with no corresponding QRS complex is helpful in determining the diagnosis of ventricular tachycardia. Lidocaine (0.25 mg/kg, IV) would be indicated in this cat.

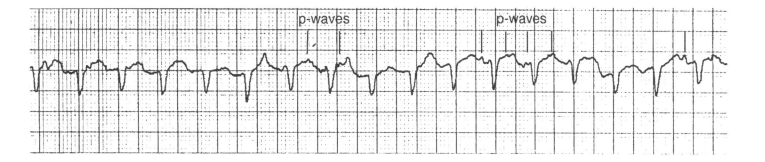

Case 16

A 4-year-old MN Boxer presents for acute syncope. Physical examination reveals a dog in good conformation and no other obvious problems. Thoracic auscultation reveals an extremely rapid and irregular heart rate and a normal pulmonary system. Femoral pulses are weak, rapid, and irregular, with many pulse deficits. An ECG is performed immediately.

Describe the arrhythmia or conduction disturbance and your approach to therapy. The answer and discussion appear on the following pages.

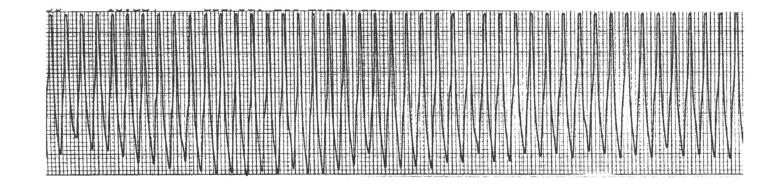

Initial Interpretation

The rhythm diagnosis is sustained ventricular tachycardia. Torsade de pointes is the specific type of sustained ventricular tachycardia.

An intravenous catheter is placed, and lidocaine (2 mg/kg, IV) or procainamide (6 mg/kg, IV) could be administered. Several minutes later, the ECG changes (lower figure).

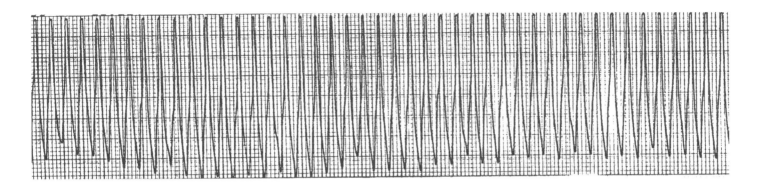

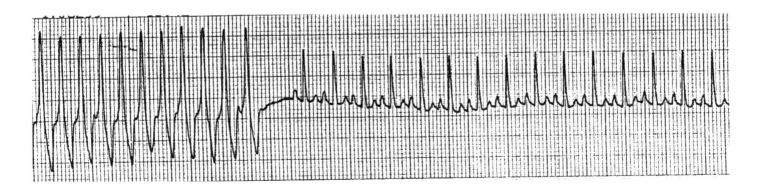

Follow-up Interpretation

The ventricular tachycardia has been converted to sinus tachycardia. There is a compensatory delay in sinus node activity following the ventricular tachycardia due to repolarization of the sinus node.

An echocardiogram is indicated to determine if this dog has underlying heart disease (dilated cardiomyopathy) or Boxer cardiomyopathy (arrhythmias only).

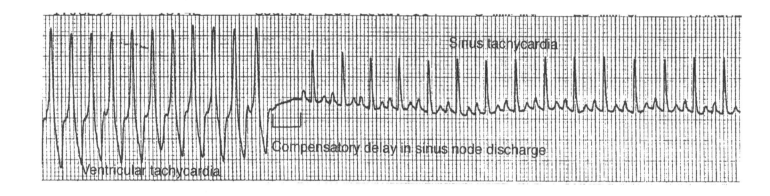

Case 17

A 10-year-old FS Poodle presents for a 4-week history of coughing that occurs primarily at night and after exercise. Otherwise, the dog has no abnormal historical findings. Physical examination reveals a grade 4/6 apical systolic murmur, heard loudest on the left hemithorax, but audible on the right hemithorax as well. Ausculta-tion also reveals irregular heart rate with occasional pulse deficits. Radiographs reveal left-sided cardiomegaly.

Describe the arrhythmia or conduction disturbance and your ap-proach to therapy. The answer and discussion appear on the follow-ing pages.

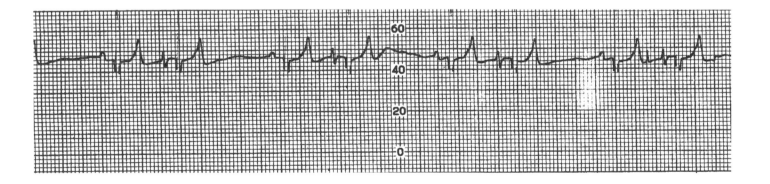

Initital Interpretation

The rhythm is sinus with atrial premature complexes occurring in a bigeminal pattern. An abnormal, premature P-wave and a normal QRS complex followed by a compensatory delay in conduction identify atrial premature complexes (circles).

Continued observation of an ECG reveals another abnormality (lower figure).

Describe the arrhythmia or conduction disturbance and your approach to therapy. The answer and discussion appear on the next page

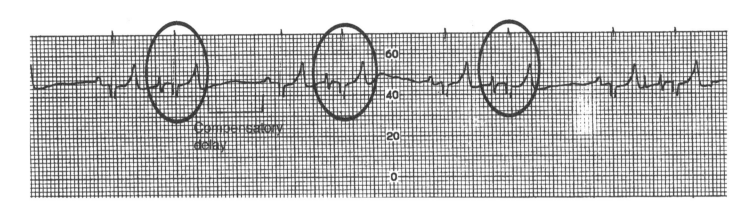

Compensatory delay

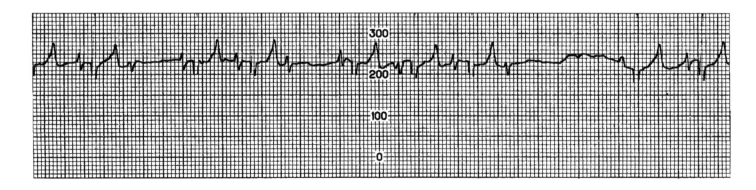

Follow-up Interpretation

A period of paroxysmal atrial tachycardia occurs at the beginning of the ECG strip with the unusual presence of a nonconducted, abnormal atrial P-wave (circles) that defines second-degree atrioventricular block. This may occur due to the refractive nature of the ventricle during the rapid rate. Therapy for atrial arrhythmias consist of slowing conduction through the AV node to allow appropriate ventricular activity with digitalis glycosides, calcium channel blockers, or beta-blockers. Therapy for the arrhythmia would not be indicated in this dog because the rhythm does not result in clinical signs of syncope or exercise intolerance.

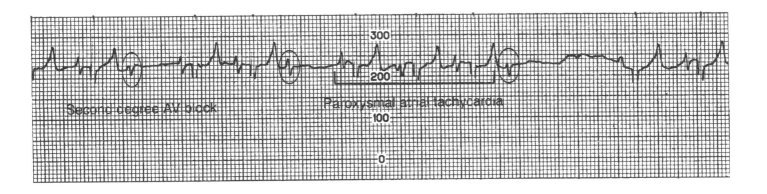

Case 18

A 14-year-old Cocker spaniel presents for episodes of syncope during exertion. Physical examination is unremarkable. Auscultation is within normal limits except for a slow, regular heart rate and femoral pulse. An ECG is performed.

Describe the arrhythmia or conduction disturbance and your approach to therapy. The answer and discussion appear on the next page.

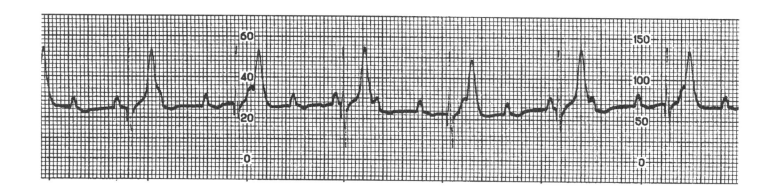

Interpretation

The rhythm diagnosis is third-degree or complete atrioventricular (AV) block. The AV node is nonfunctional in this dog and could be due to an aging change of the AV node. The sinus rate (P-waves; thin lines) is normal (120 bpm). The ventricular escape rhythm (thick lines) is 40–60 bpm. The QRS complexes do not have the typical appearance of a wide and bizarre complex. The QRS complexes appear more normal in configuration because the origin is high in the ventricle near the AV node. Definitive therapy is placement of a ventricular pacemaker.

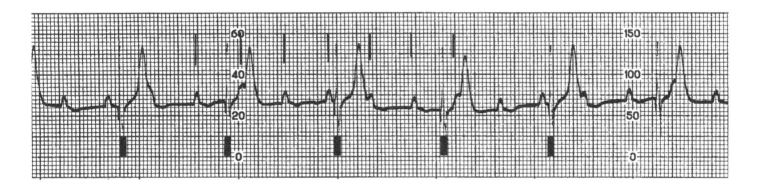

Case 19

A 4-year-old Great Dane (55 kg) presents for syncopal episodes. Physical examination reveals a very weak dog with pale mucous membranes and weak, irregular femoral pulses. Thoracic auscultation reveals a rapid, irregular heart rate and no cardiac murmur. An ECG is performed.

Describe the arrhythmia or conduction disturbance and your approach to therapy. The answer and discussion appear on the next page.

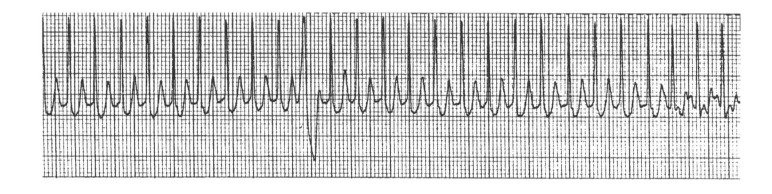

Interpretation

The ECG diagnosis is supraventricular tachycardia. The heart rate is rapid (240 bpm) and regular. The QRS complexes are normal in appearance. There is one premature ventricular complex (arrow). Primary therapy is directed to slowing the heart rate. Options include digitalis glycosides, beta-blockers (esmolol, 0.25 mg/kg, IV, slow bolus; atenolol, 0.5 mg/kg, PO), and calcium channel blockers (verapamil, 0.5 mg/kg, IV; diltiazem, 0.1 mg/kg, IV, over 5 minutes). Adenosine (0.05 mg/kg, IV, over 5 minutes) is also an option, though the effectiveness has not been determined in dogs. Primary heart disease must be ruled out as a cause of the arrhythmia. Vagal maneuvers such as compression of the globes of the eye and carotid artery massage could be attempted to increase parasympathetic tone and possibly convert the rhythm to sinus rhythm.

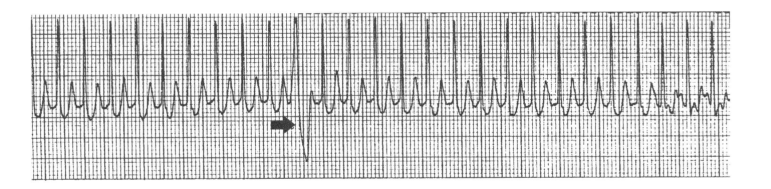

Case 20

A 12-year-old MN cat (4 kg) had a ventricular pacemaker placed several years ago for treatment of a third-degree atrioventricular (AV) block. The cat presents for acute onset of lethargy. You are able to observe the battery under the skin in the right cervicothoracic area, and it appears to be discharging properly. Auscultation reveals an irregular heart rate compared to the discharge of the battery.

Describe the arrhythmia or conduction disturbance and your approach to therapy. The answer and discussion appear on the following pages.

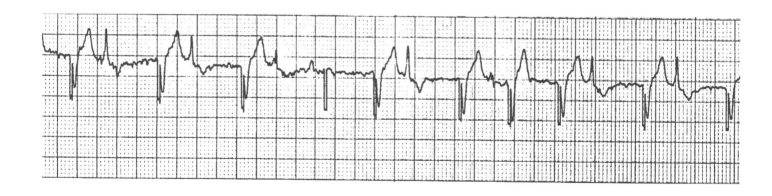

Initial Interpretation

The normal ventricular complexes generated by the pacemaker are located in the latter half of the ECG strip (stars). The pacemaker is embedded in the ventricle. Therefore, the QRS complex that is generated is ventricular in origin. Ventricular premature complexes occur immediately following a pacemaker-generated QRS complex in the beginning of the ECG strip (thick arrows), resulting in a compensatory delay in conduction. There is one pacemaker spike that does not result in a ventricular complex (thin arrow). The cat is placed on atenolol (6.25 mg, PO, SID) for control of the ventricular arrhythmias and an ECG is reevaluated in one week (lower figure).

Describe the arrhythmia or conduction disturbance and your approach to therapy.

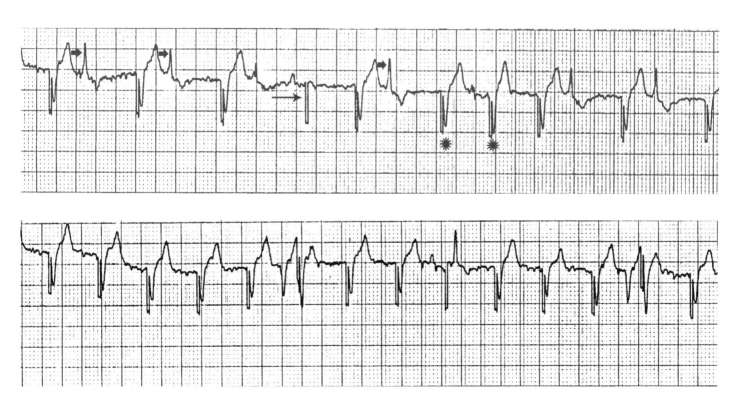

Follow-up Interpretation

There are more normal pacemaker-generated QRS complexes, with only one pacemaker spike that does not generate a complex (thin arrow). However, two pacemaker spikes (circle) occur soon after a ventricular premature complex (thick arrow). The pacemaker may not be able to detect ventricular activity and may be malfunctioning. The beginning of a pacemaker spike on the T-wave of a premature ventricular complex could lead to ventricular fibrillation. The pacemaker requires reevaluation.

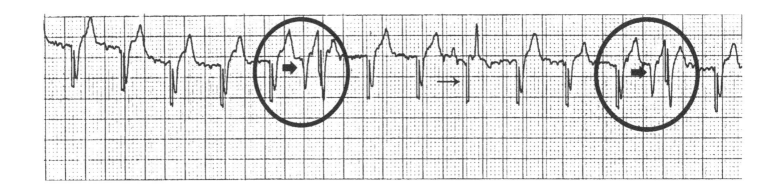

Case 21

A 7-year-old MN Doberman (35 kg) presents for a history of progressive lethargy. Physical examination reveals depression; a rapid, very weak and irregular femoral pulse; and a grade 2/6 systolic heart murmur, most prominent over the apical portion of the left hemithorax. Pulse deficits are also present and an ECG is performed.

Describe the arrhythmia or conduction disturbance and your approach to therapy.

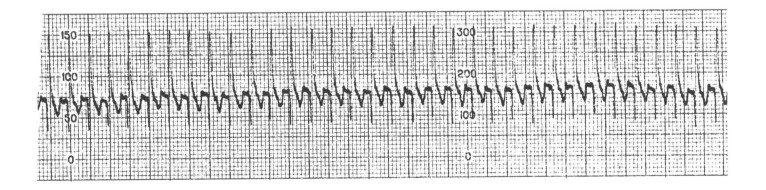

Interpretation

The rhythm is supraventricular tachycardia (SVT). The QRS complexes are normal in appearance and regular, though very rapid (290 bpm). Normal QRS complexes classify this rhythm as supraventricular in origin. It is not possible to differentiate atrial from junctional tachycardia with a rate this rapid. Atrial tachycardia is represented by the presence of abnormal P-waves. Echocardiography reveals dilated cardiomyopathy (DCM). Primary therapy for this rhythm would consist of digitalis glycosides to slow conduction through the AV node and permit slowing of the ventricular rate. Other options include calcium channel blockers (verapamil, 0.5 mg/kg, IV; diltiazem, 0.1 mg/kg, IV, over 5 minutes) and beta-blockers (atenolol, 0.5 mg/kg, PO, SID), though each can result in decreased contractility. Adenosine (0.05 mg/kg, IV, over 5 minutes) can be used in people with spontaneous occurrence of SVT (no underlying heart disease). Adenosine does not have the same success in dogs with DCM.

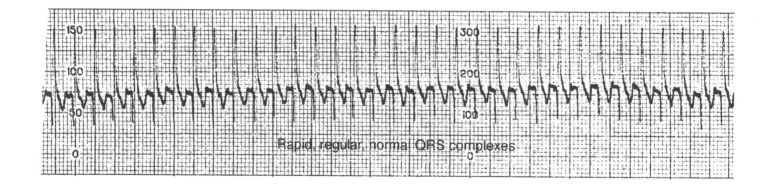

Rapid, regular, normal QRS complexes

Case 22

A 12-year-old FS Himalayan (3.5 kg) presents for evaluation of an irregular heart rhythm. The cat has a normal physical examination except for irregularity of the heart rhythm and pulse deficits. The cat is normal at home. You perform an ECG.

Describe the arrhythmia or conduction disturbance and your approach to therapy. The answer and discussion appear on the next page.

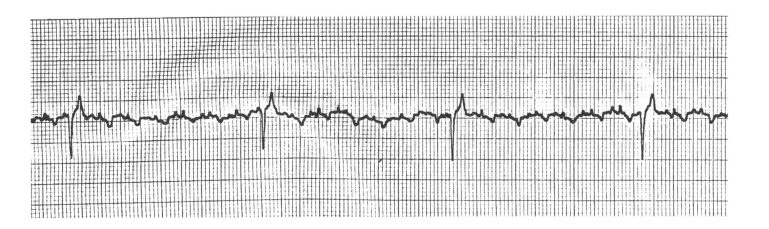

Interpretation

The rhythm is sinus with occasional premature ventricular complexes (PVCs)(thick arrows) that occur at a regular interval. Note that the P-QRS-T complexes of the normal feline ECG can be very small. A complete cardiovascular diagnostic evaluation reveals no abnormalities. The ventricular complexes are interpolated, which is described as a consistent discharge of a ventricular complex without signs of primary heart disease. Interpolated PVCs are considered benign. No therapy is indicated, though frequent reevaluations of the echocardiogram are recommended.

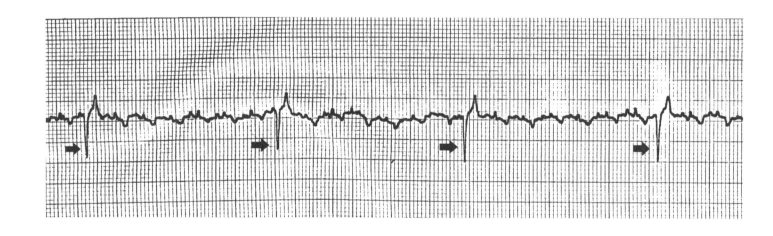

Case 23

A 6-year-old Irish wolfhound (45 kg) presents for an occasional cough and syncope. Physical examination reveals depression; rapid, slightly weak, and irregular femoral pulse; a grade 2/6 systolic murmur, most prominent over the apical portion of the left hemithorax; and multiple pulse deficits. An ECG is performed to begin the evaluation of syncope.

Describe the arrhythmia or conduction disturbance and your approach to therapy. The answer and discussion appear on the next page.

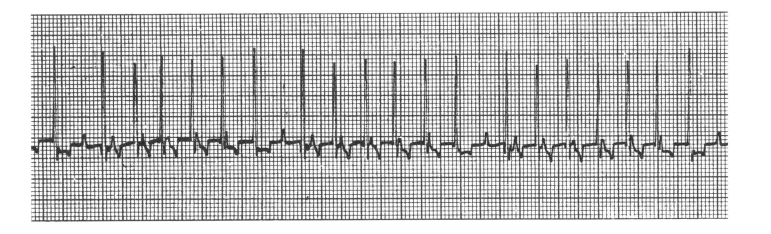

Interpretation

The rhythm is paroxysmal supraventricular tachycardia (SVT). There are occasional normal P-QRS-T complexes (circles) that are followed by short bursts (paroxysms) of SVT (bars). The normal complexes that occur are termed capture complexes, as the sinus node captures the normal rhythm. Echocardiography reveals di-lated cardiomyopathy. The rhythm is likely a prelude to the development of atrial fibrillation. Therapy would consist of slowing conduction through the AV node to allow a slower ventricular rate. Therapeutic options include digitalis glycosides, calcium channel blockers (verapamil, 0.5 mg/kg, IV; diltiazem, 0.1 mg/kg, IV, over 5 minutes), and beta-blockers (atenolol, 0.5 mg/kg, PO, SID).

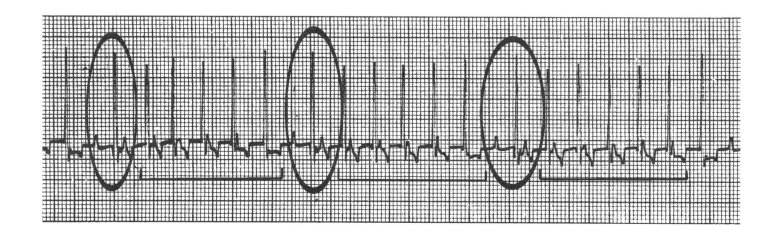

Case 24

An 8-year-old MN Maine Coon (7 kg) has been treated for hypertrophic cardiomyopathy for the last 4 years and is currently receiving diltiazem twice daily. Recently, the owner has noticed lethargy after exertion. Physical examination is unremarkable, and thoracic auscultation reveals clear lungs with a slow, regular heart rate. You perform an ECG.

Describe the arrhythmia or conduction disturbance and your approach to therapy. The answer and discussion appear on the next page.

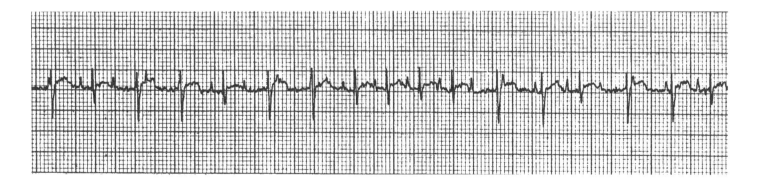

Interpretation

The rhythm is third-degree atrioventricular (AV) block. The sinus rate (thin lines) is regular and normal (180 bpm). The ventricular rate (thick lines) is regular and occurs at the normal intrinsic rate of the ventricle (160 bpm). There is no association between the sinus and ventricular complexes. The cause of the rhythm disturbance could be related to progression of the heart disease or to side effects of the diltiazem. The sinus rate is normal, so a side effect due to diltiazem is unlikely since the calcium channel blockers also can decrease sinus node discharge. The cat is not showing signs of congestive heart failure. Therapy at this point in time is not indicated. However, placement of a ventricular pacemaker may be a viable option.

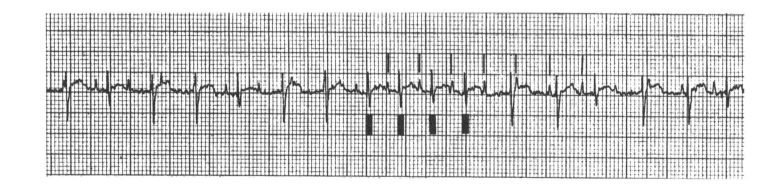

Case 25

A 13-year-old MN Persian cat (3.5 kg) has been treated for hypertrophic cardiomyopathy for the past 2 years. He is currently receiving diltiazem and enalapril. The owner has noticed that the cat is more lethargic, and a syncopal episode occurred today. Auscultation reveals a very irregular heart rate with corresponding pulse deficits. You perform an ECG.

Describe the arrhythmia or conduction disturbance and your approach to therapy. The answer and discussion appear on the following pages.

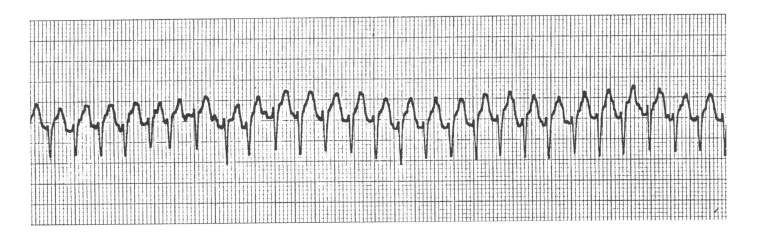

Initial Interpretation

The initial ECG diagnosis is sustained ventricular tachycardia. The QRS complexes appear abnormal in configuration, and the rate is rapid (240 bpm) and regular. Continued examination of the ECG reveals irregularity and the appearance of P-waves. A second ECG rhythm strip is examined (page 65).

Describe the arrhythmia or conduction disturbance and your approach to therapy. The answer and discussion appear on page 66.

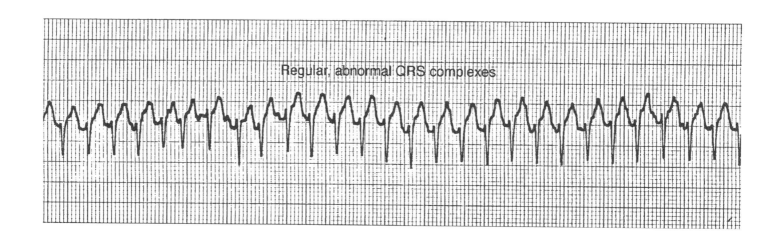

Regular, abnormal QRS complexes

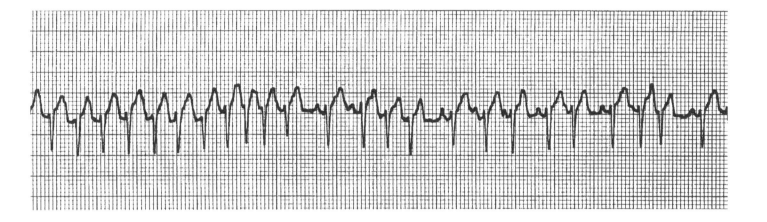

Follow-up Interpretation

Examination of the second ECG strip reveals P-waves with what appears to be a normal P-R interval and conduction through the ventricle (circles). The QRS complex does not change. Cats with hypertrophic cardiomyopathy can develop abnormal conduction through the ventricle, resulting in an abnormal appearance of the QRS complex. The conduction of the QRS complex is described as a right bundle branch block. Therefore, the tachycardia is likely junctional or supraventricular in origin. The ECG diagnosis is then described as paroxysmal supraventricular tachycardia (bars) with junctional premature complexes (thick arrow). Addition of an antiarrhythmic agent such as a beta-blocker should be considered.

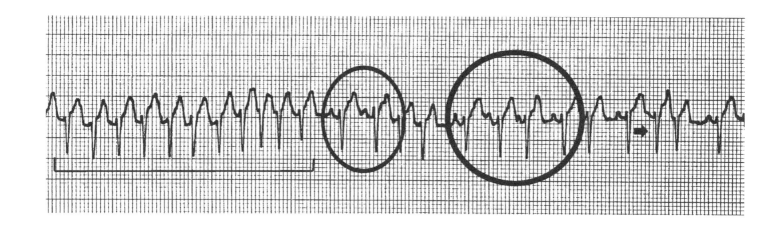

Case 26

A 12-year-old M Schnauzer (10 kg) presents for evaluation of syncopal episodes. He has been generally healthy in the past. Physical examination reveals a dog in good conformation with no obvious abnormalities. Auscultation reveals no cardiac murmur, but a very irregular rhythm with lengthy pauses. Femoral pulse is strong, yet irregular, with the same pauses noted on auscultation. An ECG is performed.

Describe the arrhythmia or conduction disturbance and your approach to therapy. The answer and discussion appear on the next page.

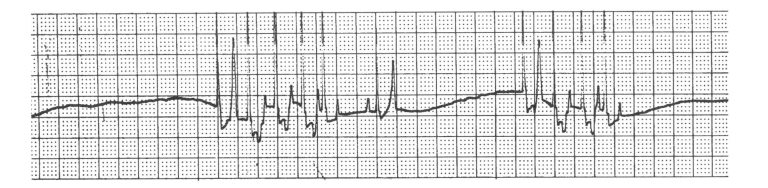

Interpretation

The primary disturbance is sinus arrest. There is a junctional escape complex (thick arrow) that is followed by paroxysmal supraventricular tachycardia (SVT) (bars). There is one normal P-QRS-T complex (circle). No antiarrhythmic therapy is indicated as the paroxysmal SVT is the rhythm that is preventing asystole and likely death. The paroxysmal SVT may also be a contraindication for atropine therapy in this dog. Definitive therapy is a transvenous atrial pacemaker.

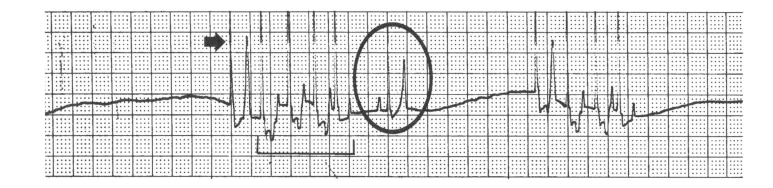

Case 27

A 10-year-old MN Australian shepherd (25 kg) presents for lethargy and exercise intolerance. Physical examination reveals jugular vein distension with jugular pulsation. Thoracic auscultation reveals normal lung sounds and rapid, muffled heart sounds. The femoral pulse is weak and rapid and an ECG is performed.

Describe the arrhythmia or conduction disturbance and your approach to therapy. The answer and discussion begin on the next page.

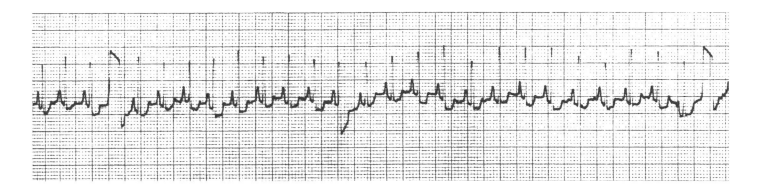

Initial Interpretation

The rhythm is sinus tachycardia with electrical alternans. The QRS complexes are smaller than normal and vary in size (circle). Pericardial effusion with tamponade should be suspected. Ultrasound reveals pericardial effusion with tamponade of the right ventricle. Pericardiocentesis is the treatment of choice.

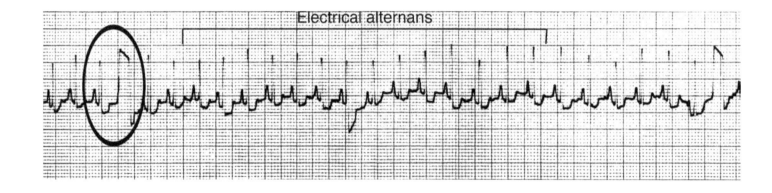

Electrical alternans

Follow-up Interpretation

Pericardiocentesis results in an immediate decrease in heart rate and respiratory sinus arrhythmia. The electrical alternans has resolved, and the QRS complex is larger (circles).

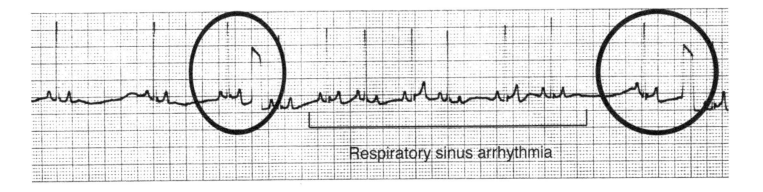

Respiratory sinus arrhythmia

Endocrine

Case 28

A 7-year-old M Samoyed (30 kg) presents for evaluation of ventricular tachycardia. Mucous membranes are pale, and the femoral pulse is weak, rapid, and irregular. Blood pressure is unable to be obtained. An ECG is performed.

Describe the arrhythmia or conduction disturbance and your approach to therapy. The answer and discussion appear on the next page.

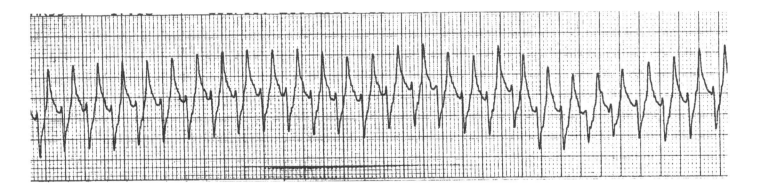

Interpretation

The rhythm diagnosis is ventricular tachycardia with a rate of 240 bpm. Fluid therapy (crystalloids and colloids) is instituted until diagnostics are completed. Electrolytes reveal hyponatremia (Na^+ = 125 mEq/L) and hyperkalemia (K^+ = 9.7 mEq/L). Addison's disease is suspected and confirmed with an ACTH stimulation test. Therapy for the ventricular tachycardia would include 10% cal-

cium gluconate (0.5–1.0 ml/kg, IV, over 10 minutes) to establish a more normal ECG. Fluid therapy and insulin (0.5 unit/kg) followed by dextrose (1–1.5 g/unit administered insulin) would also be indicated to correct the ECG. Definitive therapy for Addison's disease with fludrocortisone acetate (Florinef®) or desoxycorticosterone pivulate (Percorten®) will correct the hyperkalemia.

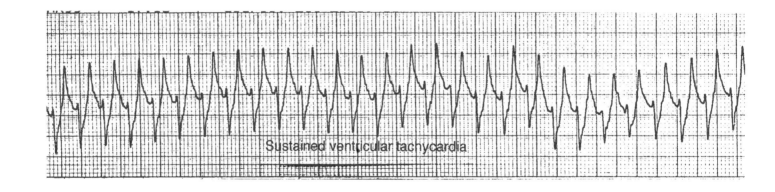

Sustained ventricular tachycardia

Case 29

A 3-year-old MN Australian shepherd (25 kg) presents in lateral recumbency. The owners report a history of vomiting and bloody diarrhea for 3 days. The owners also report a similar presentation 3 weeks ago. The dog became normal after 2 days of intravenous fluid therapy. The mucous membranes are pale, and the femoral pulse is slow and irregular. An ECG is placed as part of the initial diagnostic workup.

Describe the arrhythmia or conduction disturbance and your approach to therapy. The answer and discussion appear on the next page.

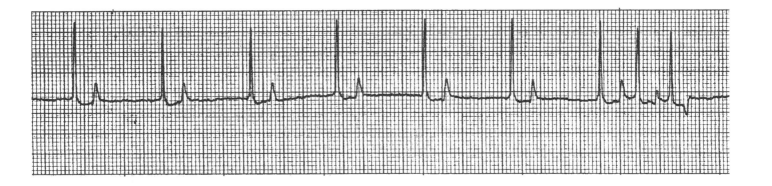

Interpretation

The rhythm is atrial standstill with junctional escape complexes (thick arrow). Two sinus complexes appear (small arrows) near the end of the ECG rhythm strip. Fluid therapy (crystalloids and colloids) is instituted until diagnostics are completed. Electrolytes reveal hyponatremia (Na^+ = 135 mEq/L) and hyperkalemia (K^+ = 11.2 mEq/L). Addison's disease is suspected and confirmed with an ACTH stimulation test. Therapy for the junctional escape rhythm should first consist of 10% calcium gluconate (0.5–1.0 ml/kg, IV, over 10 minutes) with the goal of reestablishing a more normal difference between resting membrane and threshold potential. Accomplishment of this goal will result in a more rapid heart rate. Atropine would likely be ineffective in this dog.

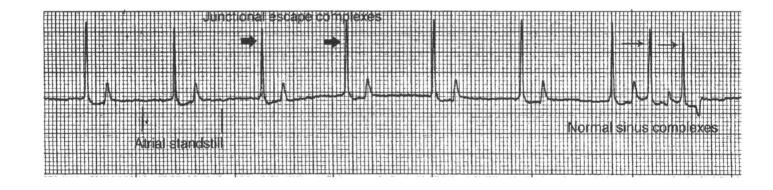

Environmental

Case 30

A 5-year-old spayed female (FS) Saint Bernard mix (65 kg) is found collapsed outdoors in subfreezing weather. The rectal temperature is below the lower limits of the thermometer (< 90°F). The dog is minimally responsive. The mucous membranes are pale, and the femoral pulse is slow, weak, and irregular. Systolic blood pressure cannot be obtained and an ECG is performed.

Describe the arrhythmia or conduction disturbance and your approach to therapy. The answer and discussion begin on the next page.

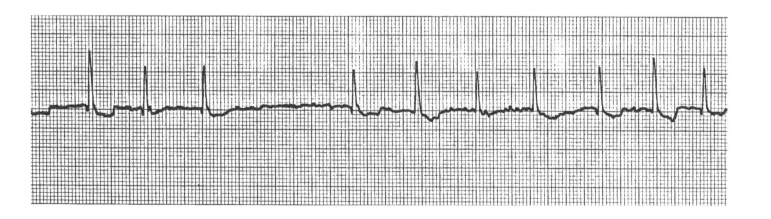

Initial Interpretation

The rhythm is atrial fibrillation. The ventricular rate is 80 bpm and irregular. There are no discernible P-waves, and the QRS complexes appear to be conducted in a normal fashion. Hypothermia can result in atrial fibrillation in people and dogs. The main difference between atrial fibrillation caused by heart disease and that caused by hypothermia is that the ventricular rate is much slower during hypothermia. A second differential diagnosis for atrial fibrillation not caused by heart disease is hypothyroidism.

The primary therapy for atrial fibrillation in this dog is aggressive external rewarming and fluid therapy with crystalloids and colloids.

Aggressive rewarming has resulted in a rectal temperature of 98°F. The femoral pulse is much stronger and remains irregular (page 83).

Describe the arrhythmia or conduction disturbance and your approach to therapy. The answer and discussion appear on page 84.

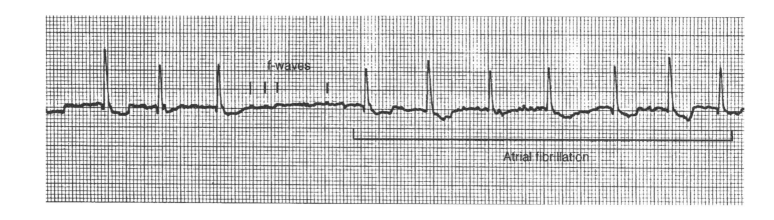

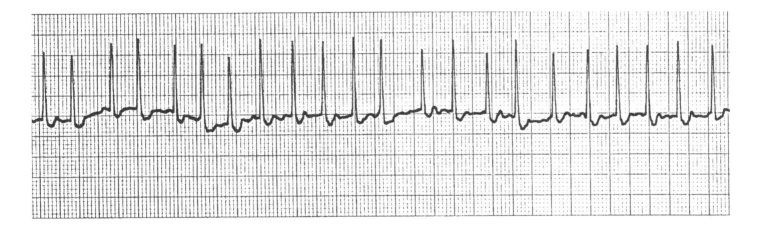

Follow-up Interpretations

The rhythm remains atrial fibrillation. The ventricular rate is higher (170 bpm) and irregular, with normal QRS complexes. There are no P-waves, although the ventricular rate appears more regular. Several hours later, the heart rate becomes more regular.

Atrial fibrillation has spontaneous converted to normal sinus rhythm (page 85). Resolution of hypothermia-induced atrial fibrillation has been reported in the dog.

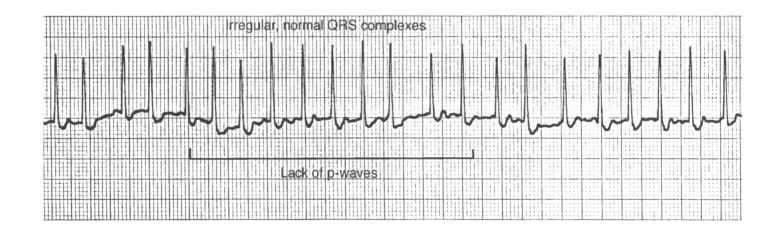

irregular, normal QRS complexes

Lack of p-waves

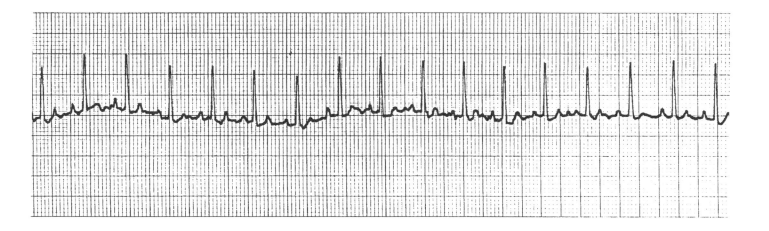

Case 31

An 8-month-old MN domestic shorthair cat (3 kg) presents after being inadvertently caught in a dryer. The owner reports that the dryer was on several minutes before the problem was recognized. The cat is extremely tachypneic, with open-mouth breathing, and the rectal temperature is 107.8°F. Indirect doppler systolic blood pressure is 50 mmHg. The heart rhythm and pulse are weak and irregular. An ECG is performed as part of the initial diagnostic plan.

Describe the arrhythmia or conduction disturbance and your approach to therapy. The answer and discussion appear on the next page.

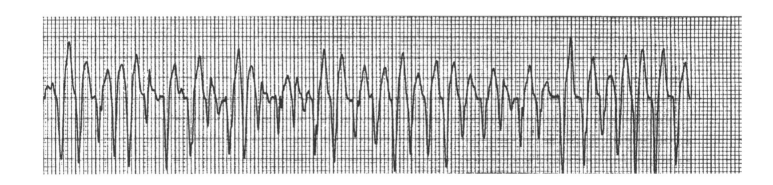

Interpretation

The rhythm is multiforme ventricular tachycardia with R-on-T phenomena (circle). All of the complexes are of ventricular origin. The various shapes of the QRS complexes (stars) indicate origins from different areas of the ventricle. Ventricular complexes arising from different areas of the ventricle imply poor perfusion to the myocardium, direct effects of hyperthermia, pain, anemia, direct trauma, acid-base disturbances, underlying heart disease, or a combination of factors. The rate is rapid (200 bpm), and overall perfusion has been affected (hypotension). The R-on-T phenomenon is a prefibrillatory event that requires immediate therapy.

The initial approach to therapy is to reestablish perfusion to the heart with oxygen by face mask or blow-by, fluid therapy with crystalloids and colloids, administration of an effective analgesic agent (hydromorphone or morphine) intravenously, and external cooling. Blood gas analysis will provide information on the acid-base status. All of the previously mentioned causes of ventricular arrhythmias need to be corrected prior to administration of an antiarrhythmic drug such as lidocaine. Potential detrimental effects of lidocaine prior to correction of the clinical abnormalities include hypotension, seizure activity, and possible worsening of the arrhythmia.

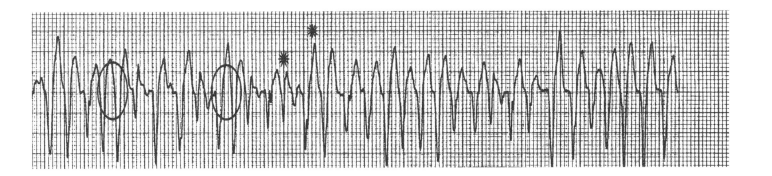

Case 32

A 12-year-old FS cat (3 kg) presents after disappearing for 4 days in very cold weather. The cat is very thin and presents in lateral recumbency. The rectal temperature does not register on your thermometer (< 90°F) and you are unable to palpate a femoral pulse. The heart rate on auscultation appears to be slow and regular. An ECG is performed.

Describe the arrhythmia or conduction disturbance and your approach to therapy. The answer and discussion appear on the next page.

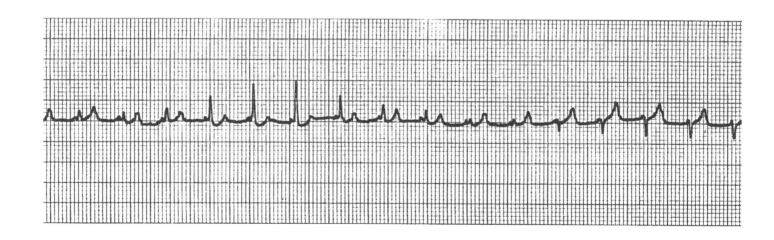

Interpretation

The rhythm is complete atrioventricular dissociation with sinus bradycardia (thin lines). There are three different ventricular foci of the QRS complexes. Hypothermia can result in decreased sinus node discharge (P-waves), atrioventricular node inactivity, and development of a ventricular escape rhythm. Primary therapy consists of external rewarming. The ECG can be reexamined after normal rectal temperature is established. Administration of an antiarrhythmic such as lidocaine is contraindicated and will likely result in termination of the ventricular escape rhythm.

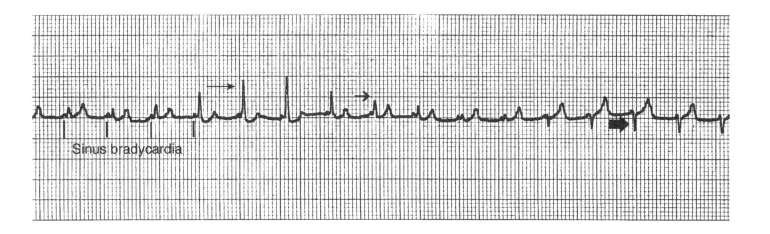

Sinus bradycardia

Case 33

A 2-year-old MN mixed breed dog (25 kg) is being treated for head trauma after being hit by a car. Adequate volume resuscitation has been established with hypertonic saline and hetastarch, based on clinical parameters of pink mucous membranes, normal capillary refill time, and blood pressure. Furosemide and mannitol were administered 3 hours previous. The initial response to fluid resuscitation and diuretic therapy was encouraging as the modified Glasgow coma score increased to a near normal value. The dog has deteriorated and is now comatose, the systolic blood pressure is 190 mmHg, and there is a very slow and irregular heart rate. An ECG is performed.

Describe the arrhythmia or conduction disturbance and your approach to therapy. The answer and discussion appear on the next page.

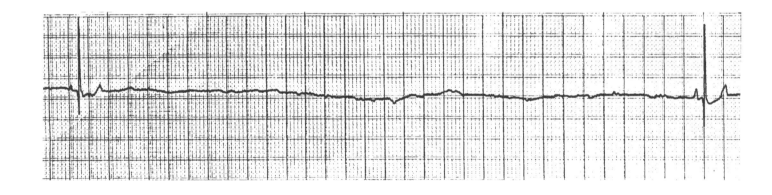

Interpretation

The primary rhythm is sinus arrest. The primary cause of the arrhythmia is likely an acute increase in intracranial pressure, possibly due to herniation of the brain. The Cushing's reflex results in hypertension and bradycardia secondary to cerebrovascular hypertension. Therapy would consist of a second administration of diuretic therapy, intubation, and ventilation. Atropine could be administered, though there is the potential for a detrimental increase in cerebral blood flow.

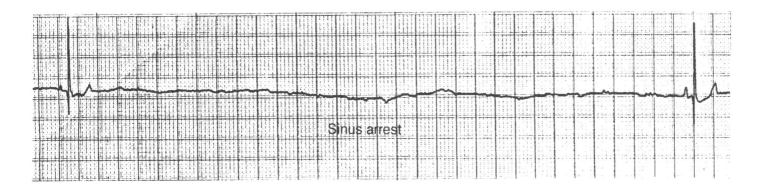

Sinus arrest

Medicine

Case 34

A 4-year-old MN Rottweiler (40 kg) presents for evaluation of chronic vomiting and is scheduled to undergo diagnostic endoscopy. Physical examination reveals a very healthy looking dog that is bright, alert, and responsive. The femoral pulse is strong but irregular. Auscultation is within normal limits except for the irregular heartbeat. Indirect blood pressure is within normal limits. An ECG is performed.

Describe the arrhythmia or conduction disturbance and your approach to therapy. The answer and discussion appear on the next page.

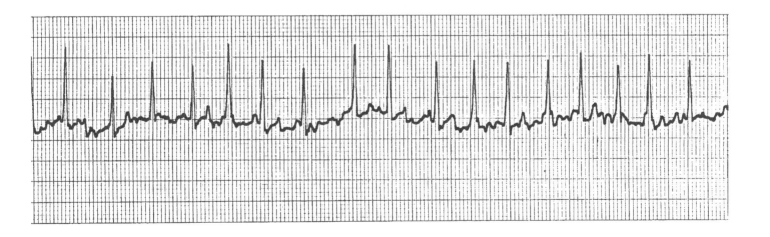

Interpretation

The rhythm is atrial fibrillation. The ventricular rate is 150 bpm and irregular, and there are fibrillation waves (thin lines). An echocardiogram is performed and is within normal limits. No antiarrhythmic therapy is indicated as the cause of the atrial fibrillation either is related to chronic intestinal disease or is considered a lone atrial fibrillation. Anesthesia consists of preanesthetic medication with diazepam (0.2 mg/kg, IM) and butorphanol (0.2 mg/kg, IM), induction with a combination of ketamine and diazepam (50:50 mixture, 1 ml/10 kg, IV; 2 ml each of diazepam and ketamine), and maintenance with isoflurane. The atrial fibrillation remains, and the heart rate and blood pressure are normal during anesthesia (page 97).

Inflammatory bowel disease is diagnosed. Prednisone (1 mg/kg PO daily) is prescribed. Two weeks later the ECG is within normal limits.

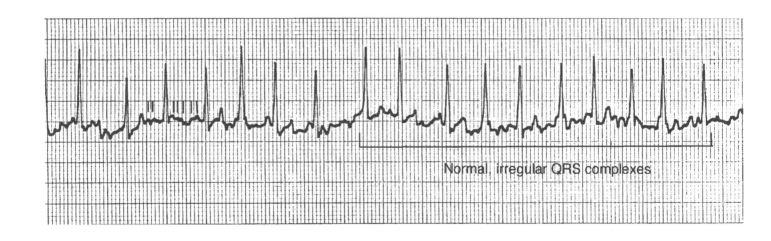

Normal, irregular QRS complexes

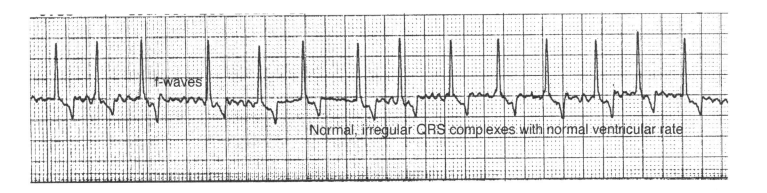

f-waves

Normal, irregular QRS complexes with normal ventricular rate

Case 35

A 10-year-old MN Maltese (5 kg) presents for acute onset of vomiting after eating chicken skin. The dog has been treated for mitral valve insufficiency for the last 3 years and is receiving enalapril (1.25 mg twice daily). Physical examination reveals a painful cranial abdomen, fever, and bile-stained vomitus. The femoral pulses are strong, rapid, and irregular. Thoracic auscultation reveals 3/6 systolic murmur and normal pulmonary sounds. Indirect systolic blood pressure is within normal limits. An ECG is performed.

Describe the arrhythmia or conduction disturbance and your approach to therapy. How will the ECG and underlying heart disease affect therapy? The answer and discussion appear on the next page.

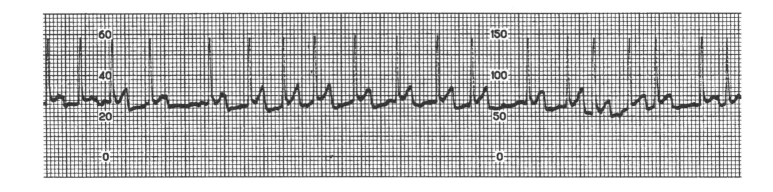

Interpretation

The rhythm diagnosis is atrial fibrillation. The ventricular rate is 180 bpm and irregular. The QRS complexes are normal in appearance. There is an absence of P-waves. The fibrillation waves that are commonly seen with atrial fibrillation are not present and have been replaced with atrial standstill.

The elevated heart rate is most likely due to pain and changes in plasma volume as a result of vomiting. The elevated heart rate is likely not a sign of cardiac decompensation due to heart disease. Fluid therapy should be administered with caution and may require invasive procedures such as central venous catheterization to monitor central venous pressure.

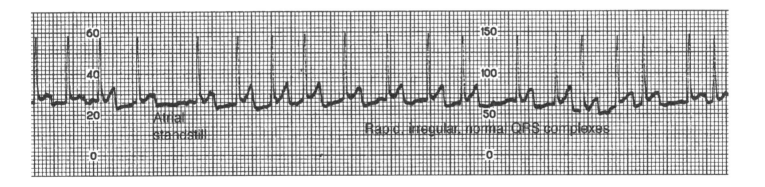

Case 36

A 10-year-old FS Siamese cat presents depressed and in lateral recumbency after a 3-week history of increased water consumption and increased urination. Mucous membranes are pale, rectal temperature is 93°F, femoral pulses are weak and irregular, thoracic auscultation is unremarkable, and the cat is hypotensive (systolic blood pressure = 50 mmHg). Initial diagnostics reveal hyper-

glycemia (blood glucose = 695 mg/dL), azotemia (creatinine = 3.4 mg/dL), and ketonuria. An ECG is performed.

Describe the arrhythmia or conduction disturbance and your approach to therapy. The answer and discussion appear on the next page.

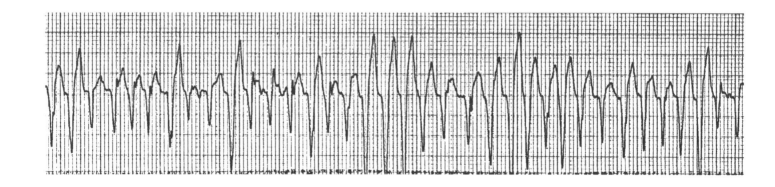

Interpretation

The ECG diagnosis is multiforme ventricular tachycardia with R-on-T phenomena (circle). The ventricular rate is 300 bpm, and there is evidence of poor perfusion (hypotension, lateral recumbency, pale mucous membranes). Immediate therapy consists of oxygen, conservative fluid therapy with crystalloids (15 ml/kg, IV) and colloids (5 ml/kg, IV), and analgesia (butorphanol, 0.2 mg/kg, IV). A decision must be made as to whether or not an antiarrhythmic agent should be administered prior to evaluation of acid-base status and electrolytes. Metabolic acidosis (poor perfusion, diabetic ketoacidosis) and hypokalemia are common causes of ventricular arrhythmias. The ECG may not respond to antiarrhythmic therapy without resolution of either abnormality. However, perfusion is poor, and the arrhythmia is considered a malignant arrhythmia. Lidocaine is administered at a low dose (0.25–0.5 mg/kg, IV). Perfusion parameters are monitored closely, external rewarming is applied, and diagnostics are performed. The arrhythmia may not improve with lidocaine therapy, and consecutive doses are not recommended until other causes of the arrhythmia are corrected.

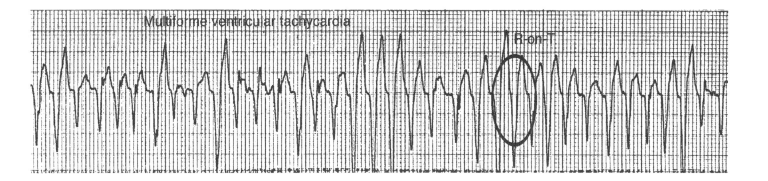

Multiforme ventricular tachycardia   R-on-T

Case 37

An 18-month-old unaltered female Chihuahua (1.5 kg) presents for evaluation of seizure activity that began at 8 weeks of age. Physical examination reveals a large, domed skull, open fontanelle, ventro-lateral strabismus of both eyes, and decreased mentation. Auscultation is normal except for a slow, irregular heart rate. The systolic doppler blood pressure is 180 mmHg, and an ECG is performed.

Describe the arrhythmia or conduction disturbance and your approach to therapy. The answer and discussion appear on the next page.

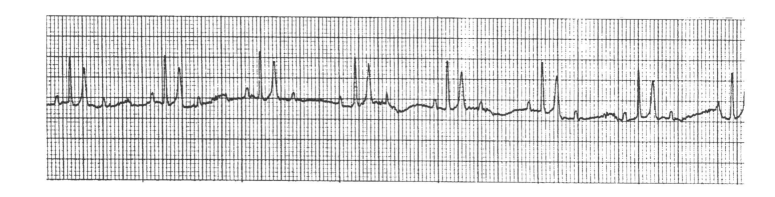

Interpretation

There is first-degree atrioventricular (AV) block (short, thin vertical line) and second-degree AV block (thick vertical line). The overall ventricular rate is slow (60 bpm), and the QRS complexes are normal. The likely cause of the arrhythmia is increased intracranial pressure resulting in systemic hypertension and bradycardia (Cushing's reflex). Primary therapy would be to decrease intracranial pressure with prednisone (decreases cerebrospinal fluid production) and furosemide. Administration of atropine could result in detrimental increases in cerebral blood flow and further increases in intracranial pressure.

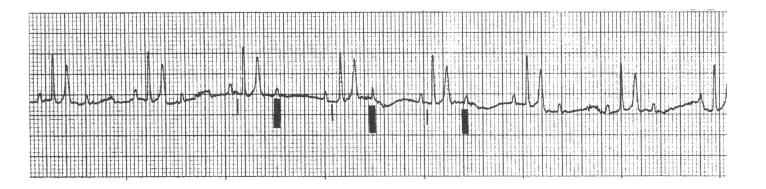

Case 38

A 2-year-old MN domestic shorthair cat (4.5 kg) presents in respiratory distress. There has been a long history of asthma, and therapy has consisted of prednisone as needed for an acute crisis. The cat is currently not receiving prednisone. The cat is open-mouth breathing with an increased inspiratory effort and an exaggerated expiratory effort. Expiratory wheezes are auscultated, and there is no heart murmur. Mucous membranes are cyanotic. Oxygen ad-

ministration results in some improvement of the respiratory distress, though mucous membranes are minimally improved. The femoral pulse is slow and irregular.

Describe the arrhythmia or conduction disturbance and your approach to therapy. The answer and discussion appear on the next page.

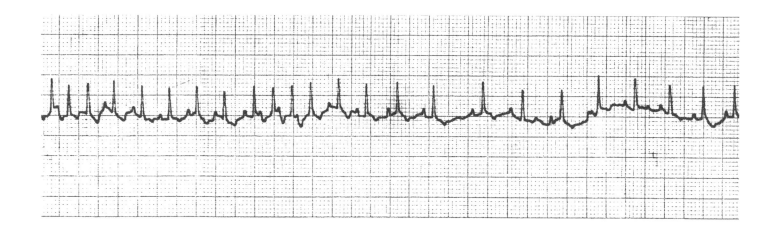

Interpretation

The rhythm is sinus bradycardia with paroxysmal junctional tachycardia (circle). The bradycardia is likely due to severe hypoxemia. The junctional arrhythmias are also likely due to hypoxemia and myocardial tissue hypoxia. Primary therapy is to provide oxygenation. Capturing the airway by intubation may be required. Antiarrhythmic drugs are unlikely to be effective without adequate oxygenation.

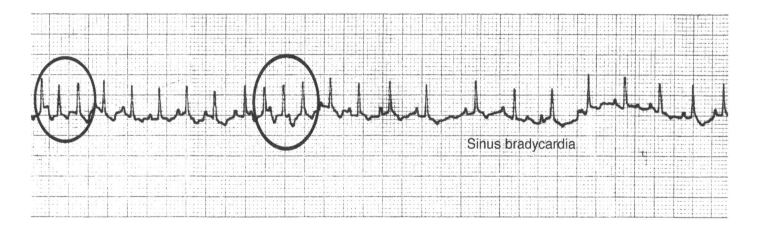

Sinus bradycardia

Perioperative

Case 39

A 7-year-old MN Great Dane (50 kg) is being monitored for 24 hours following surgery to correct a gastric dilatation-volvulus (GDV). Anesthesia and surgery were uncomplicated. A continuous ECG is being monitored during the postoperative period. The technician observes what appears to be an abnormality.

Describe the arrhythmia or conduction disturbance and your approach to therapy. The answer and discussion appear on the next page.

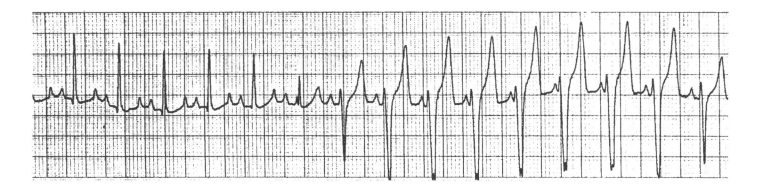

Interpretation

The ECG begins as sinus rhythm with a heart rate of 110 bpm. An accelerated ventricular rhythm appears in the latter half of the ECG tracing with a ventricular rate of 110 bpm. Fusion complexes (arrows) occur prior to the accelerated ventricular rhythm. A fusion complex is described as a complex that is the combination of the normal sinus complex and the ventricular complex. A fusion complex has no clinical significance, and no therapy is required. The accelerated ventricular rhythm occurs at a rate that is very similar to the normal sinus rate.

Gastric dilatation-volvulus is a multisystemic disorder that can result in several disorders that predispose the heart to ventricular arrhythmias. These include

- poor perfusion resulting in tissue hypoxia, reperfusion injury, and metabolic acidosis;

- acid-base disturbances including metabolic and respiratory acidosis;

- electrolyte disturbances such and hypokalemia and hypo-magnesemia;

- anemia due to blood loss;

- pain; and

- primary heart disease.

A decision on the need for antiarrhythmic therapy is based on the collection of clinical and laboratory data. Therapy is usually not warranted if clinical and laboratory values are normal. An accelerated ventricular rate below 150–170 bpm does not require antiarrhythmic therapy. The accelerated ventricular rhythm with a rate similar to the sinus rate typically results in normal cardiac output and a clinically normal patient.

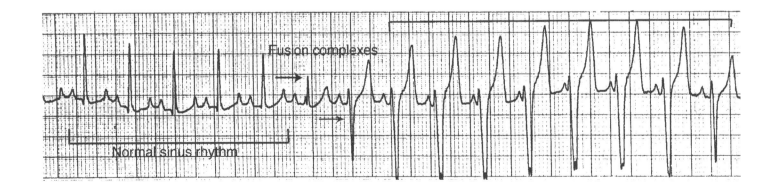

Fusion complexes

Normal sinus rhythm

Case 40

A 5-year-old MN Bulldog (20 kg) is recovering from an entero-tomy performed the previous day to remove a foreign object. Hydromorphone (0.1 mg/kg, IV; 2 mg; every 4 hours) is being administered for postoperative analgesia, and the dog is resting comfortably. The technician notes that the heart rate is slower than the previous day and is more irregular. An ECG is performed.

Describe the arrhythmia or conduction disturbance and your approach to therapy. The answer and discussion appear on the next page.

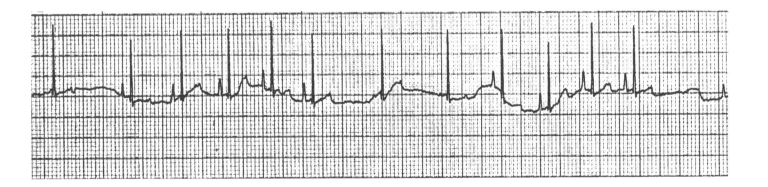

Interpretation

The rhythm is respiratory sinus arrhythmia. There are junctional escape complexes (arrows) that occur during the expiratory phase of respiration. The heart rate increases during inspiration and decreases during expiration due to normal parasympathetic responses. Hydromorphone is an opioid agonist that can increase parasympathetic tone and exacerbate the respiratory sinus arrhythmia. The escape complexes are identical in appearance to the normal QRS complexes. Therefore, the origin of the escape complexes is in or very close to the atrioventricular node. No therapy is warranted in this dog. Clinical parameters of perfusion (mucous membranes, blood pressure, femoral pulse) indicate no detrimental effect of the arrhythmia on the cardiovascular system. Administration of a parasympatholytic agent (atropine or glycopyrrolate) could result in sinus tachycardia and the possibility of tachyarrhythmias.

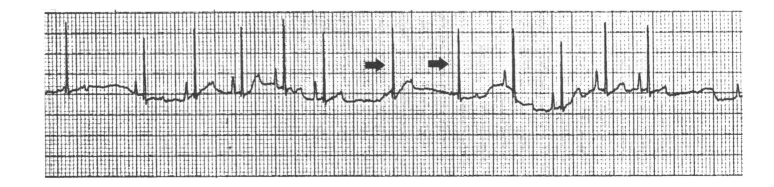

Case 41

A 10-year-old FS Golden retriever is being monitored after having a splenectomy. The dog presented in severe hemorrhagic shock. Initial stabilization was with hypotensive resuscitation using het-astarch (5 ml/kg) and lactated Ringer's solutiuon (LRS) (45 ml/kg) intravenously until the systolic blood pressure was above 60 mmHg. The dog was hypotensive throughout anesthesia despite therapy with Oxyglobin® (4 ml/kg, IV bolus) during surgery. The dog is currently receiving a whole blood transfusion. Vital signs at the time of the ECG include hypotension (indirect Doppler systolic blood pressure = 75 mmHg), pale mucous membranes, and a rapid, irregular, and weak femoral pulse.

Describe the arrhythmia or conduction disturbance and your approach to therapy. The answer and discussion appear on the next page.

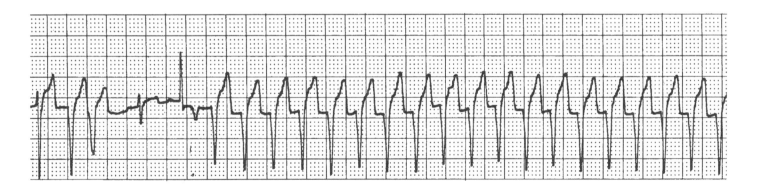

Interpretation

The rhythm is multiforme ventricular tachycardia with R-on-T phenomena (circle) that progresses to sustained ventricular tachycardia. Hypotension may be the primary factor in the development of this arrhythmia. Hypotension could be due to continued bleeding, anemia, reperfusion injury, pain, electrolyte disturbances, or a combination of factors. A jugular venous catheter should be placed to monitor central venous pressure (CVP), which would provide information regarding the intravascular volume status. Once CVP is determined, decisions could be made regarding the use of antiarrhythmic drugs. Administration of lidocaine or procainamide in a patient with poor volume could result in severe hypotension.

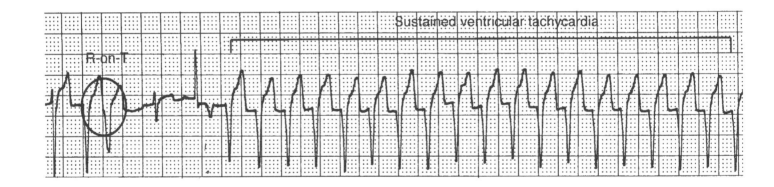

Case 42

A 6-year-old FS Bull mastiff presents for nonproductive vomiting and abdominal distension of 4–6 hours duration. Initial diagnosis is gastric dilatation-volvulus and is confirmed with a right lateral radiograph. Indirect systolic blood pressure is low (60 mmHg), mucous membranes are pale, and the femoral pulse is weak and irregular. An ECG is performed.

Describe the arrhythmia or conduction disturbance and your approach to therapy. The answer and discussion appear on the next page.

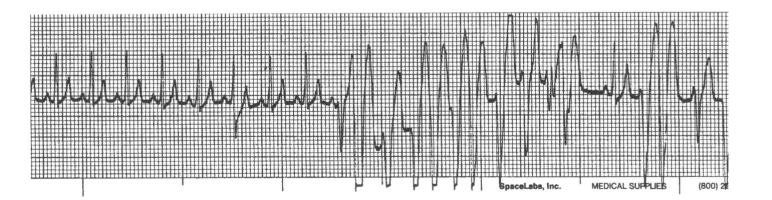

SpaceLabs, Inc.   MEDICAL SUPPLIES   (800) 2

Interpretation

The ECG begins with sinus tachycardia and proceeds to paroxysmal multiforme ventricular tachycardia with R-on-T phenomena (small circle). The causes of sinus tachycardia followed by the ventricular arrhythmia in this dog include hypotension as a result of obstruction of venous return, blood loss, pain, electrolyte disturbances (low potassium), acid-base disturbances (metabolic acidosis), and hypoxemia secondary to ventilation perfusion imbalances as a result of the distended abdomen. Therapy includes oxygen, correction of hypotension (fluid support), decompression of the distended stomach, and analgesia (opioid agonist) prior to the administration of antiarrhythmic drugs. Administration of lidocaine or procainamide could result in worsening of the hypotension if there is not adequate intravascular volume.

There are two areas of artifact on the ECG related to movement of the patient (arrow and large oval). The movement artifact during paroxysmal multiforme tachycardia has resulted in the complexes being cut off at the bottom of the ECG strip.

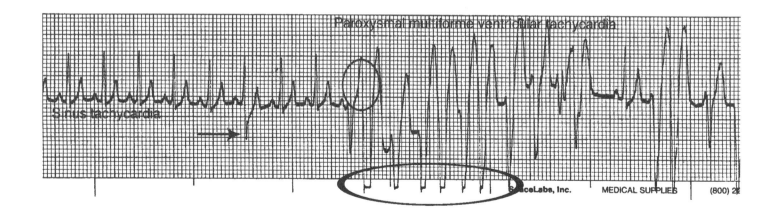

Case 43

A 9-year-old MN Labrador retriever is being monitored 12 hours after successful surgery to correct a gastric dilatation-volvulus. A continuous ECG has been monitored since the end of surgery, and abnormalities are noticed. Physical examination reveals the dog is more pale than normal, especially during the arrhythmia.

Describe the arrhythmia or conduction disturbance and your approach to therapy. The answer and discussion appear on the next page.

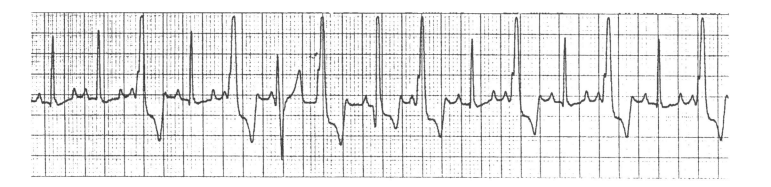

Interpretation

Multiforme premature ventricular complexes (arrows) occur with a sinus rhythm (circles). Several diagnostic tests are necessary to determine the approach to therapy. Gastric dilatation-volvulus is a multisystemic disorder that can result in several abnormalities that can predispose the heart to ventricular arrhythmias including

- poor perfusion resulting in tissue hypoxia, reperfusion injury, and metabolic acidosis;
- acid-base disturbances including metabolic and respiratory acidosis;
- electrolyte disturbances such and hypokalemia and hypomagnesemia;
- anemia due to blood loss;
- pain; and
- primary heart disease.

Laboratory results for this dog reveal normal packed cell volume and total solids, adequate analgesia, and normal arterial and central venous blood gas. Electrolytes reveal hypokalemia (2.6 mEq/L) and normal magnesium.

Hypokalemia can result in ventricular arrhythmias and should be corrected with potassium supplementation prior to administration of antiarrhtyhmic agents.

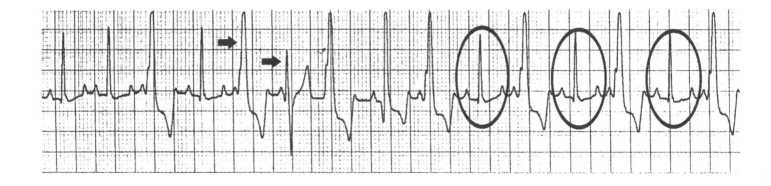

Case 44

An 8-year-old MN Rottweiler (45 kg) is being monitored following successful splenectomy. A large splenic mass with no evidence of bleeding was found on physical examination after a presentation of anorexia, lethargy, and occasional vomiting for the past 3 days. Anesthesia and surgery were uneventful, and an ECG has been monitored since the end of surgery 2 hours previous. Analgesia consists of intermittent butorphanol administration. Clinical pa-

rameters including blood pressure (110 mmHg systolic) and mucous membrane color with capillary refill time (pale/pink, 2 seconds) are within normal limits. The dog is uncomfortable in the cage and changes positions often.

Describe the arrhythmia or conduction disturbance and your approach to therapy. The answer and discussion appear on the next page.

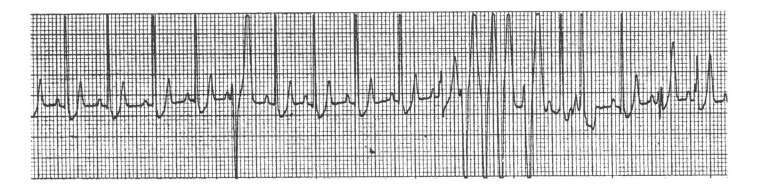

Interpretation

The rhythm is sinus with one premature ventricular complex (thin arrow) and a fusion complex (thick arrow) followed by paroxysmal ventricular tachycardia. The paroxysmal ventricular tachycardia is very rapid and contains R-on-T complexes (circle).

Several problems soon after splenic surgery can predispose the heart to ventricular arrhythmias. These include

- poor perfusion from postoperative blood loss, which can result in myocardial tissue hypoxia, reperfusion injury, and metabolic acidosis;
- pain;
- anemia;
- acid-base disturbances including metabolic and respiratory acidosis;
- electrolyte disturbances such and hypokalemia and hypo-magnesemia; and
- primary heart disease.

Immediate therapy with lidocaine (2 mg/kg, IV bolus) would be indicated due to the rapid ventricular rate and R-on-T complexes and normal cardiovascular parameters.

Physical examination reveals inadequate analgesia. Butorphanol is an opioid agonist-antagonist with mild to moderate analgesia. A more potent opioid such as hydromorphone (0.1 mg/kg, IV, every 4 hours) should be administered. Reassessment of analgesia should commence prior to the continued administration of lidocaine or other antiarrhythmic agents.

All other laboratory diagnostics were within normal limits.

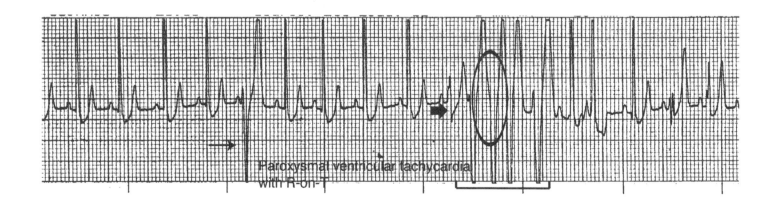

Paroxysmal ventricular tachycardia with R-on-T

Case 45

A 2-year-old FS Great Dane (40 kg) is being monitored 16 hours after successful surgery to correct a gastric dilatation-volvulus. A continuous ECG has been monitored since the end of surgery, and today you notice some abnormalities. The dog has a normal physical examination, pink mucous membranes with a capillary refill time of 2 seconds, and Doppler systolic blood pressure of 120 mmHg.

Describe the arrhythmia or conduction disturbance and your approach to therapy. The answer and discussion appear on the next page.

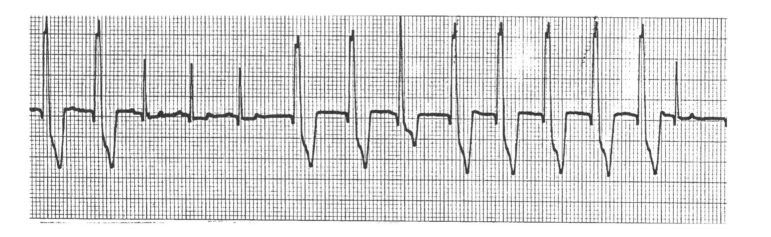

Interpretation

There is sinus rhythm with an accelerated ventricular rhythm. The rate of the sinus rhythm and ventricular rhythm is similar and normal. There is no physical evidence of perfusion abnormalities. Gastric dilatation-volvulus is a multisystemic disorder that can result in several disorders that predispose the heart to ventricular arrhythmias. These include

- poor perfusion resulting in tissue hypoxia, reperfusion injury, and metabolic acidosis;
- acid-base disturbances including metabolic and respiratory acidosis;
- electrolyte disturbances such and hypokalemia and hypomagnesemia;
- anemia due to blood loss;
- pain; and
- primary heart disease.

Determination of the causes of ventricular arrhythmias will reveal the approach to therapy. All laboratory tests are normal. There is no indication for antiarrhythmic therapy in this dog unless the heart rate increases or the ventricular complexes become multiform or more rapid. Most accelerated ventricular rhythms do not require therapy unless the rate is above 150–170 bpm or there is a clinical effect as a result of the arrhythmia (poor perfusion).

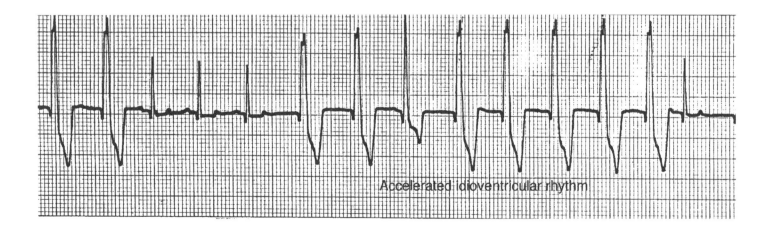

Accelerated idioventricular rhythm

Case 46

A 15-year-old FS Shih Tzu (6 kg) is recovering from a thoracotomy to perform a right pneumonectomy. Surgery and anesthesia were uncomplicated. Analgesia consists of intrapleural bupivacaine, transdermal fentanyl, and an infusion of morphine, lidocaine, and ketamine. Blood pressure is normal, mucous membranes are pink, and respirations are normal. The ECG appears abnormal.

Describe the arrhythmia or conduction disturbance and your approach to therapy. The answer and discussion appear on the next page.

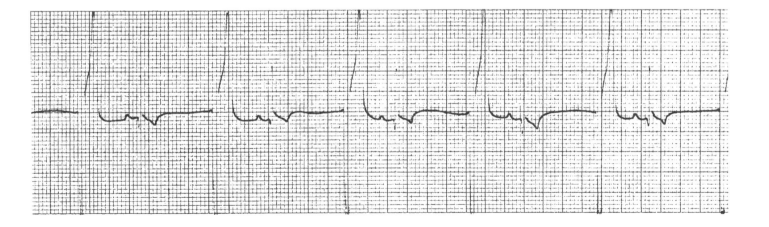

Interpretation

The ECG diagnosis sinus bradycardia that results in ventricular escape complexes (thick arrows). Therapy would consist of arousing the dog to determine if the escape complexes resolve as the heart rate increases. Atropine could be administered if the sinus rate decreased and hemodynamics became abnormal, indicating poor perfusion. Antiarrhythmic therapy with lidocaine or procainamide is not indicated and could be detrimental.

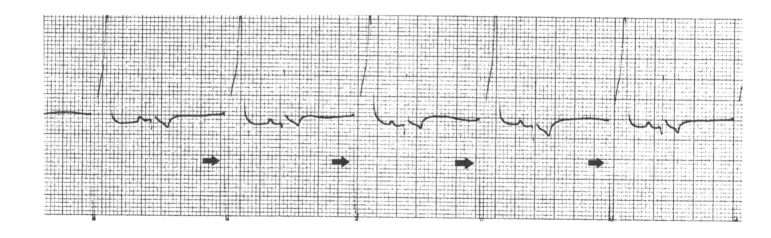

Renal

Case 47

A 1-year-old MN domestic shorthair cat (5 kg) presents in lateral recumbency. The owners report that the cat has been going in and out of the litter box for 3 days. A large, firm bladder is palpated. The femoral pulse is slow and regular, and an ECG is placed.

Describe the arrhythmia or conduction disturbance and your approach to therapy. The answer and discussion appear on the next page.

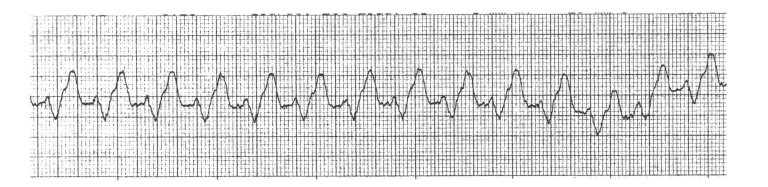

Interpretation

The ECG depicts an extremely slow idioventricular rhythm. The QRS complexes are described as sinusoidal in appearance. Hyperkalemia should be suspected. The potassium of this cat (12.1 mEq/L) is very high, and intravenous calcium gluconate therapy (0.5–1 ml/kg, IV, over 5 minutes) should be administered immediately. Calcium will reestablish the normal difference between resting membrane and threshold potential that potassium has narrowed. Therefore, the action potential can act in a more normal fashion until the potassium can be lowered. Administration of insulin (1 unit) followed immediately by 50% dextrose (5 ml) will drive potassium into the cell. Fluid therapy will also decrease the potassium. Calcium gluconate, insulin and dextrose, and fluid therapy should commence prior to placing a urethral catheter.

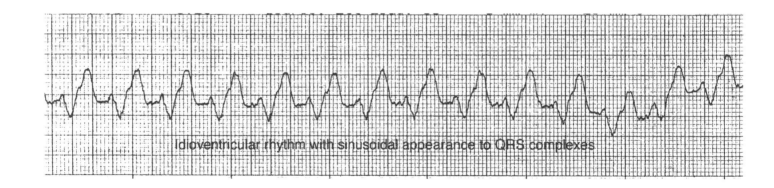

Idioventricular rhythm with sinusoidal appearance to QRS complexes

Case 48

A 5-year-old MN domestic shorthair cat (5.5 kg) presents for inability to urinate. The owners report that the cat has been going in and out of the litter box for 3 days. A large, firm bladder is palpated. The cat is depressed but aware of its surroundings. The femoral pulse is regular, and an ECG is placed.

Describe the arrhythmia or conduction disturbance and your approach to therapy. The answer and discussion appear on the next page.

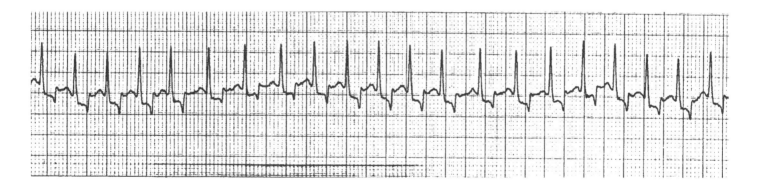

Interpretation

The rhythm is normal sinus rhythm with a normal rate of 180 bpm. Electrolytes reveal hyperkalemia (K^+ = 7.5 mEq/L). Hyperkalemia does not necessarily produce expected ECG changes in every patient, as there are multiple factors involved with generation of the ECG other than potassium concentration. Sedation or anesthesia in a patient with hyperkalemia and a normal ECG could still result in detrimental effects if the potassium is not decreased prior to the administration of anesthetic drugs.

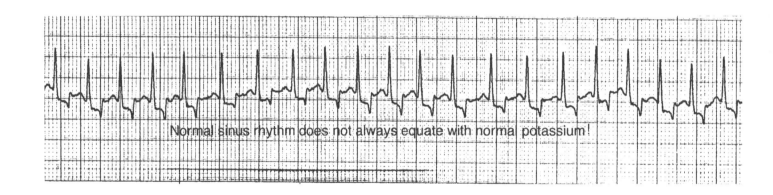

Normal sinus rhythm does not always equate with normal potassium!

Trauma

Case 49

A 2-year-old MN Labrador retriever (45 kg) presents immediately after being hit by a car. The owner reports that the dog has had difficulty breathing since the accident. Physical examination reveals severe respiratory distress with muffled pulmonary and cardiac sounds. Blood is being expelled from the nose and mouth. Oxygen by mask is administered. An ECG is placed as venous access is obtained.

Describe the arrhythmia or conduction disturbance and your approach to therapy. The answer and discussion appear on the following pages.

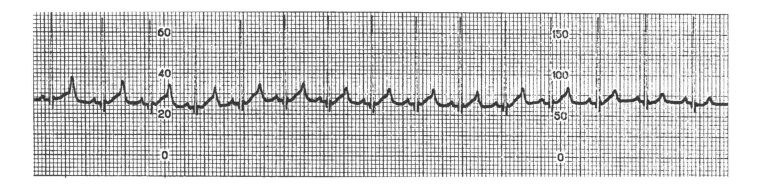

Initial Interpretation

The rhythm is sinus tachycardia. Potential causes include hypoxemia secondary to pulmonary contusions and/or pneumothorax, hypovolemia (relative or absolute), or pain.

The dog's condition worsens as fluid therapy is being administered. The respiratory rate has slowed, and the mucous membranes have become cyanotic. The ECG has also changed dramatically (lower figure).

Describe the arrhythmia or conduction disturbance and your approach to therapy. The answer and discussion appear on the next page.

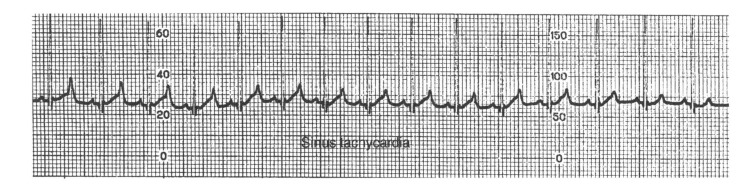

Sinus tachycardia

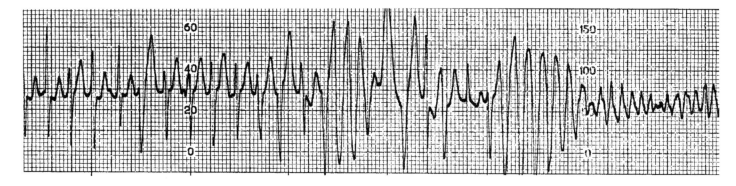

Follow-up Interpretation

The rhythm is multiforme sustained ventricular tachycardia with R-on-T phenomena (circles). The second episode of R-on-T results in ventricular fibrillation and cessation of respirations. Intubation and open-chest cardiopulmonary resuscitation (CPR) is indicated immediately. The injury to the thorax may be revealed and be relieved upon entering the chest. Closed-chest CPR would be much less effective in this dog.

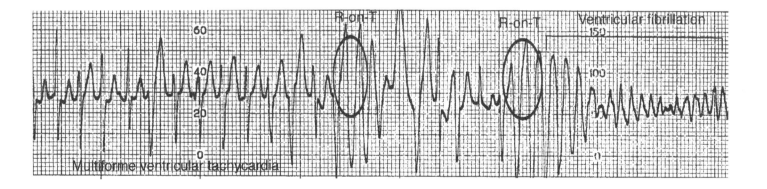

Case 50

A 2-year-old male cat (5 kg) presents after being attacked by two dogs. The cat is recumbent with an open fracture of the right radius. Mucous membranes are pale, no femoral pulse is palpated, and the cat is hypothermic. You place an ECG and begin resuscitative therapy.

Describe the arrhythmia or conduction disturbance and your approach to therapy. The answer and discussion appear on the next page.

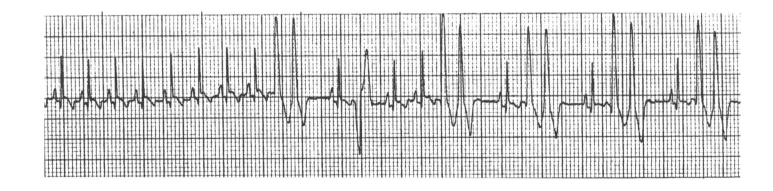

Interpretation

The rhythm begins as sinus tachycardia (240 bpm). Several multiforme ventricular premature complexes occur (arrows), and there are several episodes of R-on-T (circle).

Intravenous analgesia (hydromorphone, 0.1 mg/kg) is administered as the arrhythmias could be result of pain or may be exacerbated by pain. Intravascular volume therapy is instituted on a conservative basis during external rewarming by using crystalloids (15 ml/kg, IV) and colloids (5 ml/kg, IV). The decision to administer an antiarrhythmic agent is made after rewarming and reassessment of the cardiovascular status. Immediate administration of an antiarrhythmic agent such as lidocaine could result in hypotension.

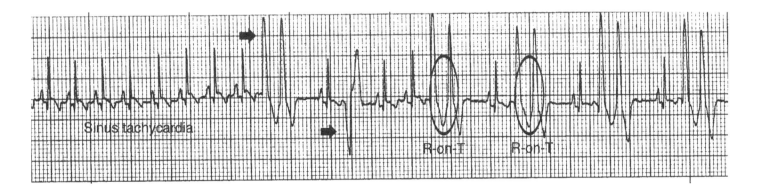

Sinus tachycardia   R-on-T   R-on-T

Case 51

A 15-month-old F mixed-breed dog (15 kg) is being treated for injuries associated with being hit by a car. There is a simple, closed, left tibial fracture that has been splinted. Initial signs of shock were successfully treated with colloids and analgesia. A continuous rate infusion (CRI) of morphine (0.12 mg/kg/hr) is being administered, and a transdermal fentanyl patch (25 μg/kg/hr)has been placed. The technician notes that while the dog is sleeping the heart rate decreases, and there appear to be pauses in the rhythm. The blood pressure is normal, and the mucous membranes are pink with a capillary refill time of 2 seconds. The femoral pulse is strong, yet irregular. There are no pulse deficits. Continuous ECG is being monitored by telemetry.

Describe the arrhythmia or conduction disturbance and your approach to therapy. The answer and discussion begin on the next page.

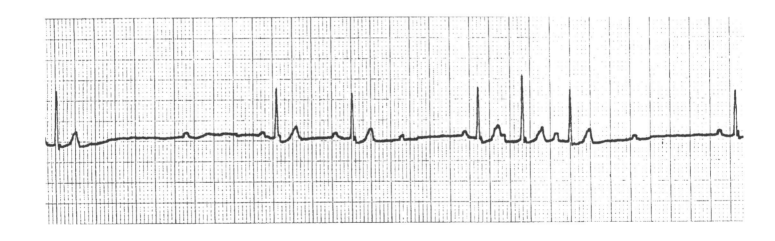

Initial Interpretation

The underlying rhythm is respiratory sinus arrhythmia as the sinus rate (P-waves) increases and decreases with respiration. The P-R interval is prolonged (bars) and is described as first-degree atrioventricular (AV) block. There are occasional P-waves with no corresponding QRS complex (thin line), which defines second-degree AV block. There is one junctional escape complex (thick arrow) that occurs after a nonconducted P-wave.

The dog awakens as the cage door is opened. The ECG is noted to become more regular (page 140).

Describe the arrhythmia or conduction disturbance and your approach to therapy. The answer and discussion appear on page 141.

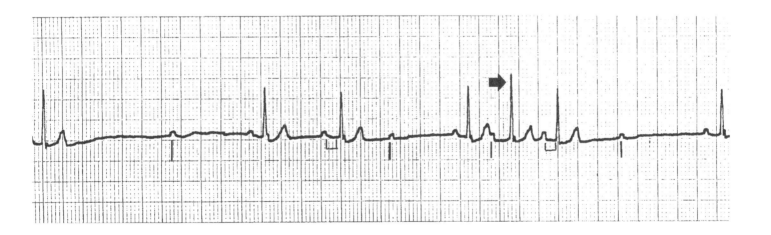

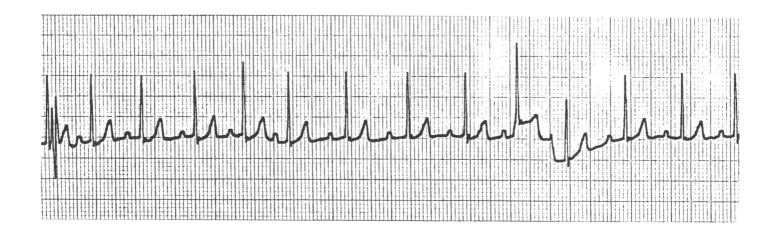

Follow-up Interpretation

The overall rhythm is normal sinus rhythm. The first-degree AV block persists (bars), and there is a movement artifact (circle). The second-degree block has resolved. The scenario is common with continuous rate infusion of opioids in stable animals. The morphine can decrease sinus node discharge and can exacerbate respiratory sinus arrhythmia as a result of increased parasympathetic tone. Second-degree AV block can also occur. Sleep can intensify the effects of the morphine. Mild stimulation (awakening) results in a relative increase in sympathetic tone. The result is an increase in sinus node discharge and resolution of the second-degree AV block (increased conduction though the AV node). No therapy is warranted because hemodynamic variables are normal during the arrhythmia. Atropine could be administered as the dog sleeps. However, an increase in heart rate could result in unnecessary increased myocardial work.

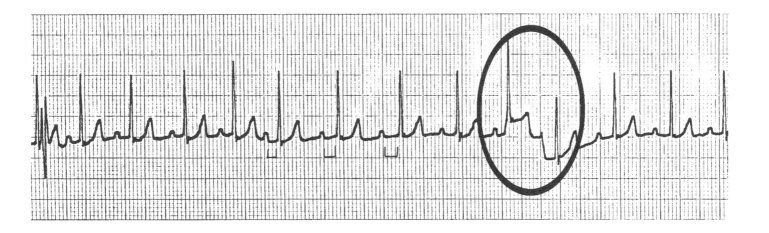

Case 52

A 6-week-old M kitten (1 kg) presents after being found outside in the snow. The kitten is recumbent and has a rectal temperature that does not register on the thermometer (< 90°F). The heart is difficult to auscultate, and a femoral pulse is not palpated. Blood pressure is unable to be obtained.

Describe the arrhythmia or conduction disturbance and your approach to therapy. The answer and discussion appear on the next page.

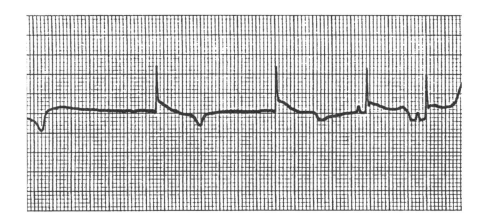

Interpretation

The rhythm is periods of sinus arrest with junctional escape complexes (thick arrows). There are two P-waves that appear to conduct to the ventricle in a normal fashion (circle). The Q-T interval (bars) is prolonged as a result of hypothermia. Hypothermia results in decreased electrical activity of the heart. Atropine administration would be ineffective for therapy of this rhythm as increased parasympathetic tone is not the cause of the conduction disturbance. Aggressive external and internal warming is indicated as the primary therapy.

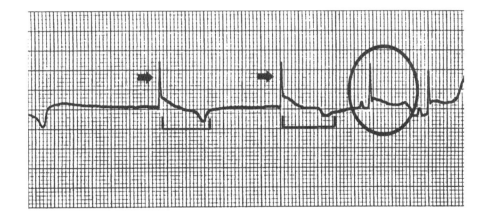

Case 53

A 6-year-old MN Labrador retriever (30 kg) presents after being hit by a car. Initial hemodynamic parameters included hypotension, tachycardia, pale mucous membranes, and weak femoral pulse. Physical examination revealed a fracture of the left femur. Initial resuscitation consisted of oxygen, hetastarch, and analgesia with butorphanol (0.2 mg/kg, IV). Hemodynamic parameters improved with initial therapy, and the dog appears to be stable. Continuous ECG monitoring 2 hours later reveals an abnormality.

Describe the arrhythmia or conduction disturbance and your approach to therapy. The answer and discussion appear on the next page.

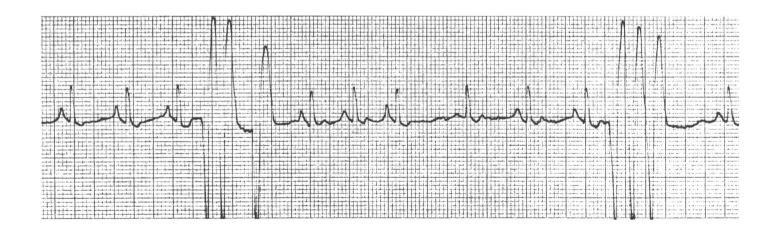

Interpretation

The underlying rhythm is respiratory sinus arrhythmia. Paroxysmal ventricular tachycardia (circles) occurs with R-on-T phenomena. Trauma can result in several disorders that predispose the heart to ventricular arrhythmias. These include

- poor perfusion resulting in tissue hypoxia, reperfusion injury, and metabolic acidosis;

- anemia due to blood loss (internal or at the fracture site);

- pain (inadequate analgesia);

- acid-base disturbances including metabolic acidosis;

- electrolyte disturbances such and hypokalemia and hypomagnesemia; and

- primary heart disease.

Determination of the causes of ventricular arrhythmias will reveal the approach to therapy. Laboratory tests do not reveal severe bleeding, blood gas examination is normal, and hemodynamic parameters are normal.

Analgesia for a femoral fracture should consist of more potent agents than butorphanol. Administration of an opioid agonist such as morphine as a continuous rate infusion (with or without lidocaine and ketamine), administration of an intermittent bolus of morphine or hydromorphone, and addition of a potent nonsteroidal anti-inflammatory agent would be recommended prior to administration of an antiarrhythmic agent. If analgesia were assessed to be normal, then administration of an antiarrhythmic such as lidocaine (2 mg/kg, IV) or procainamide (6 mg/kg, IV) would be warranted.

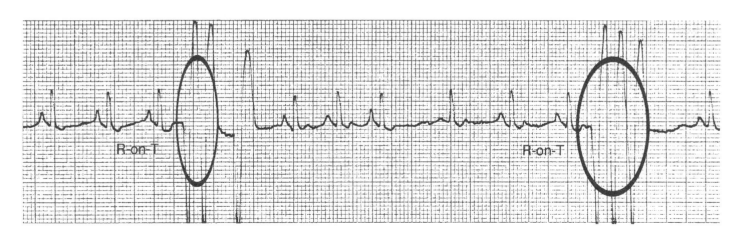

Index